Breast Cancer
The Unplanned Journey
Lessons Learned

Breast Cancer
The Unplanned Journey
Lessons Learned

Beverly Stacy Dittmer

COPYRIGHT © 2011 BY BEVERLY STACY DITTMER.

LIBRARY OF CONGRESS CONTROL NUMBER:		2011911743
ISBN:	HARDCOVER	978-1-4628-4877-5
	SOFTCOVER	978-1-4628-4876-8
	EBOOK	978-1-4628-4878-2

All rights reserved. No part of this book may be reproduced or transmitted in any form or by any means, electronic or mechanical, including photocopying, recording, or by any information storage and retrieval system, without permission in writing from the copyright owner.

Some of the names of the real people in this book have been changed. The medical statements in this book are only what I understood and are not to be taken as true medical facts. One should always obtain exact medical information from a qualified and licensed medical representative. Also be aware that the treatment of Cancer changes and gets better daily. My knowledge was obtained in 2003 and 2004.

The illustrations for the cover of this book were done by Liz Dittmer.

This book was printed in the United States of America.

COVER DESIGNED BY LIZ DITTMER

To order additional copies of this book, contact:
Xlibris Corporation
1-888-795-4274
www.Xlibris.com
Orders@Xlibris.com
97632

Contents

Introduction—It Is CANCER 17

Chapter 1-Facing the Worst Makes the Problem Seem Smaller 19
    A. General Facts about Me 19
    B. The Summer Devastation of 2002 20
    C. A Typical Week in My Life (Before I Knew I Had Cancer) 21
        1. Durango Activities.. 21
        2. White-Water Rafting 22
        3. Friends 23
        4. Family 24
    D. Last Outing Before Cancer 24
    E. Finding "the Lump" 25
        1. Self-Breast Exam that Was Different 25
        2. Sandy's Breast Cancer 26
    F. Learning to Live with "the Lump" 26
        1. Living One Day at a Time 26
        2. Accepting the Worst 27

Chapter 2-Everything Moves So Slowly 29
    A. Diagnosing 29
        1. First Appointment with Nurse Practitioner 29
        2. Mammogram 29
        3. Passing the Time Waiting 30
        4. Sonogram 31
        5. Surgeon's Appointment 31
    B. Accepting My Condition 31

Chapter 3-Make the Journey One Step at a Time 33
    A. Meeting My Surgeon 33
    B. Passing the Time 34
        1. Off to Texas 34
        2. Back to Durango with Two Grandchildren 34
    C. The Lumpectomy 34

    D. After the Surgery 36
    E. Cancer for Sure 36
        1. The Doctor Called 36
        2. Telling My Family and Friends 37
        3. Living the First Night with "the Monster" 38
    F. Hibernating 39
    G. Waiting to See the Surgeon Again 40

Chapter 4-Ask Questions, Find Answers 42

Chapter 5-Use Others' Support, But Watch Out for the Negative 46
    A. Waiting for Another Surgery 46
    B. Support from All 47
    C. A Very Sad, Bad Cancer Tale 47
    D. Just Getting By 48

Chapter 6-Life and Plans Go On—Go with the Flow 50
    A. Another Surgery 50
    B. Hosting My High School Class Reunion 51
    C. Monday, July 28, from My Diary 52

Chapter 7-Follow the Doctor's Directions, Especially In Pain Management 54
    A. Pain Management 54
    B. Surgery Recovery 55
    C. More Bad News 56

Chapter 8-Carefully Keep Your Records—Medical and Personal 57
    A. Medical Records 57
    B. Your Personal Support Records 58

Chapter 9-Find Good Models—Cancer Survivors 60

Chapter 10-Store Memories of Strength and Happiness 62
    A. MD Anderson Appointment 62
    B. Last-Minute Tasks 63
        1. Hopes and Help 63
        2. My Writing E-mail Lists 63
    C. Getting Ready to Leave 64
        1. Doctor's Release 64
        2. Shutting Down the Colorado Home 64
        3. Saying Good-bye 65
        4. My Breast Condition 65
        5. Final Plans 66
    D. The Departure Day Arrived, Leaving Colorado 66
    E. Staying at Mary Lee's House 66
    F. Joining the World of the Living Again 67

Chapter 11-Listen to Your Body 68
    A. Life in Grapevine, Texas 68
        1. Breaking a Solid Board with My hand............................ 68
        2. The Consequences of My Not Listening to My Body 70
    B. Treating This New Condition.. 71
        1. The Long, Dreary Drive Back to Grapevine 71
        2. A Saturday Morning Very Early in the ER................................. 72
        3. More Lessons Learned 74
    C. Recovering Again.. 74

Chapter 12-Patience—Fighting Cancer Is Not a Race 76
    A. The Trip to Houston 76
    B. MD Anderson.. 77
        1. A Reputable Cancer Hospital 77
        2. What Took Me So Long to Get to MD Anderson 77
    C. Keeping the First Appointment.. 79
        1. Finding the Facility.. 79
        2. Seeing the Doctor 79

Chapter 13-The Journey Can Be Full of Unexpected Turns—Just Go On......... 81
    A. Preparing for Clean-out Surgery... 81
    B. Third Surgery.. 82
    C. Recovery Room Trial 82
    D. Healing at MD Anderson Hospital 83
    E. What Was My Clean-out Surgery 83
    F. Hospital Boredom 84
    G. Going Home in Houston to Heal 85
        1. A Restful Sunday 85
        2. Monday—A Test Day 85
        3. Tuesday, Going Back Just to Get the Gauze Changed 86
    H. Later in the Week at MD Anderson 87

Chapter 14-The Decision-Making Committee Is A Necessity..................... 88
    A. My Medical Decision Committee... 88
    B. Another Lumpectomy or a Mastectomy?.................................... 89
    C. A Single or a Double Mastectomy? 89

Chapter 15-Keep Reminders of Love and Support with You 91
    A. My Yellow Comfort Bag 91
    B. The Special Heart Pillow 92

Chapter 16-Good News along the Journey!—
Seeing a Light at the End of the Unplanned Journey 93
    A. After-Surgery Checkup.. 93

        1. Test Results 93
        2. Double Mastectomy Plans.. 93
        3. My Feelings about the Planned Surgery 94
   B. The Unplanned Journey Education Continued 95

Chapter 17-The Darkest Time 97

Chapter 18-Use All Resources 99
   A. Returning to MD Anderson 99
   B. The Unplanned Journey—Living Fully with Cancer" 99
        1. Breakout Session "Rest and Relaxation"—Inner Mind Symbols
           Reflect Your Life 100
        2. Breakout Session "Journaling"—Communicate
           Your Inner Fears and Feelings 101
           a. I'm From 102
           b. Cancer Personified.. 103
           c. Dark Times 104
        3. Breakout Session "Taming Your Inner Dragons" 105
        4. Friday Morning Speakers 105
           a. John Mendelsohn.. 105
           b. Bob Arnot 105
           c. Ted Kennedy 106
        5. Roundtable Discussions 106
        6. Breakout Session "Am I Done Yet?" 107
        7. Breakout Session "Health Profiles of Cancer Survivors" 107
        8. Breakout Session "Chemobrain: Cognitive Impairment" 107
        9. Breakout Session "Coping with the Fear of Reoccurrence" 108
        10. Friday Evening Banquet 108
        11. Talk by a Comedian Entitled
           "Don't Look Back—We're Not Going that Way" 108
        12. Survival Panel Discussion 109
        13. Breakout Session "Breakthroughs in the Treatment of Breast
           Cancer".. 109
        14. Survivors' Birthday Party 110
        15. My Learnings from This Seminar 110

Chapter 19-Completing All My "Before Surgery"
Tasks—Waiting with the Monster 112
   A. My Physical Condition at This Time 112
   B. Seeing My Mother Again... 112
   C. Seeing Lilli.. 113
   D. Going Back to Colorado 114

    E. Bev's Boobs' Begone Bash 115
    F. Talking to John... 117
    G. Unexpected, Unplanned Illness.. 117
    H. The Last Day in Grapevine, Saturday, September 13 118
    I. Sunday September 14, 2003, the Last Day of My Sabbatical............... 120

Chapter 20-Gather Your Support Team.. 122
    A. My Support Staff 122
    B. Thanks to My Companion 122
    C. Thanks to My Doctor Daughter 123

Chapter 21-Private Feelings 124
    A. My Very Private Thoughts 124
    B. Going to the Hospital.. 126

Chapter 22-Suppressing Your Fears 128
    A. Waking Up with Seemingly Real Monsters............................. 128
    B. Mary Joy's Presence Brings Rationality 129

Chapter 23-Concentrate on the Important Things 131
    A. Settling Down to Recover 131
    B. My First Day After Surgery 132
    C. Saying Good-bye to My Doctor Daughter 132
    D. Seeing My Mastectomy Sites.. 133
    E. Talking to the Anesthesiologist about My Nightmares............. 133
    F. Laughter Enters My Hospital Room 133
    G. Going Home to Spring.. 135

Chapter 24-The Real Bottom 137
    A. Recovery 137
    B. A Bump in the Road 138
    C. The Good News Comes 139

Chapter 25-Don't Go It Alone... 141
    A. Returning Home 141
    B. Another Setback.. 142
    C. The Hospital Again 143

Chapter 26-Hard Times Are Relative—Remember Job from the Bible? 146
    A. Home Again from the Hospital... 146
    B. Earlier Hard Times.. 146
    C. My Cancer—The Next Hard Time 147
    D. Another Crisis 147
    E. My Job Time 148
    F. My Fluid Collection... 148
    G. Back to MD Anderson 149

Chapter 27-Getting Ready for Chemotherapy 151
    A. Finding Out about My Chemo 151
    B. My Chances of Getting Breast Cancer Again 151
    C. American Cancer Society Help 152
    D. Chemotherapy "How To" Class 152
    E. Moving to Houston 153

Chapter 28-Taxol Chemo Treatments 154
    A. Chemo to Begin 154
    B. Settling In 154
    C. My First Chemo Treatment 155
    D. Living with Chemo 155
    E. Draw a Chart of Your Task Time 156

Chapter 29-Bald and Beautiful 158
    A. Second Treatment 158
    B. Third Treatment 158
    C. Passing the Time between Treatments 159
    D. Thoughts about Chemo from My Letters 159
    E. Side Effects Already 160
    F. A Rude Awakening—The Bill 162
    G. My Marriage Anniversary and "Normal" Life 162
    H. My Fourth Chemo Treatment 164
        1. Bad Weather 164
        2. Underarm Drainage 164
        3. Healing Hands 164
        4. Actual Chemo Treatment 165
        5. Best Week Ever 166

Chapter 30-Let the Chemo Kill My Cancer 168
    A. Taxol Treatment Number Five 168
        1. Central Line Catheter Reinsertion 168
        2. Chemo Treatment 169
        3. Thanksgiving Day, 2003 169
        4. Sores and Lesions and Extreme Fatigue 170
    B. Sixth Chemo Treatment 171
        1. Chemo Treatment and Life 171
        2. My Birthday 172
        3. Head Sore Updates and My Current Appearance 173
        4. Life Continues On 174

Chapter 31-The End of a Bad Year 176
        A.   Treatment Number Seven 176
        B.   Treatment Number Eight 176
        C.   Christmas at MD Anderson and At Our Apartment 177
        D.   Stolen Bikes 178
        E.   Treatment Number Nine 179
        F.   Christmas In Grapevine 179
        G.   A Time of Contemplation 180

Chapter 32-Halfway Done 186
        A.   The New Year, 2004 186
        B.   Treatment Number 11 186
        C.   Twelfth and Last Taxol Chemo Treatment 187

Chapter 33-Count My Blessings—I'm Alive 190
        A.   I Meet the Red Devil 190
        B.   Hesitation and Fears 191
        C.   FAC Treatment Number One 191
        D.   At Home with the Adriamycin Pump 192
        E.   Back to the Hospital for the Final Infusions 194
        F.   Thoughts about Cancer 195
        G.   Alive to Go On 196

Chapter 34-Keeping on Keeping On 198
        A.   A Time between Treatments 198
        B.   FAC Treatment a Second Time 199
        C.   Food and FAC 201
        D.   Holiday Celebrations 201
        E.   Fingernail and Toenail Infections 202
        F.   Neuropathy 202
        G.   Thoughts on Taking the Next Treatment 204
        H.   Trip Back to Grapevine 205
        I.   MD Anderson Thoughts 206
        J.   Valentine Wishes for My Family and Friends 206

Chapter 35-The End of the Journey 208
        A.   The Third Treatment and Finally, New Hair 208
        B.   Finally, New Hair 208
        C.   Fourth FAC Treatment 209
              1.   Blood Count Too Low 209
              2.   Friends Come to Help Pass the Weekend 209
              3.   Finally I Get the Last FAC Treatment 209

	D. The Natural High (written 4:10 a.m. early Thursday)	210
	E. Beginning Life Again	211
	F. Quitting Lexapro	212
	G. Healing from Final Treatment	212
Chapter 36-Normal Life Is Good		**214**
	A. Normal Life Wasn't Easy	214
	B. Good-bye to Houston	214
	C. Final Activities	215
	D. Houston in Our Rearview Mirror	216
	E. My Last Cancer Report	217
	F. Making the Wishes Come True	217

The Unplanned Journey Time Line

May 20, 2003	Left Texas and journeyed to Durango, Colorado
June 10, 2003	Found a lump in my right breast.
June 18, 2003	Appointment with Nurse Practitioner
June 18, 2003	Mammogram in Durango
June 24, 2003	Sonogram in Durango
July 2, 2003	Appointment with Surgeon, Dr. Dwight Dover
July 3, 2003	Left Durango to go to family reunion in Texas
July 8, 2003	Returned to Durango with two grandchildren
July 9, 2003	Pre-op appointment with Dr. Dwight Dover
July 11, 2003	First lumpectomy in Durango
July 15, 2003	Doctor calls with results from path report. I have Cancer
July 17, 2003	Another appointment with doctor to decide what to do
July 21, 2003	Second lumpectomy and Sentinel Node Biopsey
July 25, 2003	McCamey High School Class Reunion began at my house
July 28, 2003	McCamey High School Class Reunion ended at my house
July 29, 2003	Received path report. Cancer had spread. No clear margins
July 30, 2003	Appointment to see Dr. Dover and obtain release to go to Texas, drain tubes come out
August 5. 2003	Left Colorado to travel back to Texas
August 6, 2003	Beverly, Paul, and Mr. Boots arrive at the Texas house
August 7, 2003	BeautiControl Conference and breaking the board
August 8, 2003	My right breast explodes
August 14, 2003	Appointment at MD Anderson, Clean-out surgery
August 21, 2003	Follow-up visit to Dr. Ralston
August 22, 2003	Travel back to Grapevine
August 26, 2003	Visit Mother and Sister in Coleman
September 3, 2003	Back to MD Anderson, Houston
September 5 – 7, 2003	The Unplanned Journey Seminar
September 7, 2003	Trip back to Colorado to visit
September 9, 2003	Bev's Boobs Begone Bash
September 10, 2003	Return to Grapevine

September 13, 2003	Birthday party for MJ
September 14, 2003	Back to Houston to see kids
September 15, 2003	Double Mastectomy Surgery
September 17, 2003	Home to Spring
September 20, 2003	ER at MD Anderson
September 24, 2003	Return home to Grapevine
September 30, 2003	ER at Grapevine, Texas
October 6, 2003	Home again in Grapevine
October 9, 2003	Drain tubes removed
October 14, 2003	Return to MD Anderson with drainage collection under my arms
October 15, 2003	Meet oncologist and make chemotherapy plans
October 21, 2003	Move to Houston
October 22, 2003	Back to MD Anderson to see Dr. Brawn and others
October 27, 2003	First Chemo Treatment
November 3, 2003	Second Chemo Treatment
November 10, 2003	Third Chemo Treatment
November 17, 2003	Fourth Chemo Treatment
November 18, 2003	First trip home to Grapevine
November 24, 2003	Fifth Chemo Treatment
November 27, 2003	Thanksgiving Day
December 1, 2003	Sixth Chemo Treatment
December 4, 2003	My sixty first birthday
December 8, 2003	Seventh Chemo Treatment
December 15, 2003	Eighth chemo treatment
December 22, 2003	Ninth chemo treatment
January 5, 2004	Eleventh chemo treatment
January 12, 2004	Twelfth and last Taxol chemo treatment
January 21, 2004	First FAC treatment
February 11, 2004	Second FAC treatment
March 3, 2004	Trip to Grapevine to see Erica swim
March 8, 2004	Third FAC treatment
March 29, 2004	Scheduled fourth FAC treatment
April 5, 2004	Fourth FAC treatment
April 9, 2004	Go to Grapevine
April 11, 2004	Easter
April 16, 2004	Return to Houston
April 22, 2004	Last appointment at MD Anderson
April 24, 2004	Hauled furniture and miscellaneous to sell at the resale shop
April 30, 2004	Left Houston for good
December, 2009	Finished writing *Breast Cancer—The Unplanned Journey*

Breast Cancer

The Unplanned Journey
Lessons Learned

Beverly Stacy Dittmer

Introduction

IT IS CANCER

What does one do at six thirty in the evening, when your surgeon calls to inform you that the results of your pathology report are finally in and that your lump was Cancer? My world and everything in it all of a sudden came crashing down. Time stood still. It was as if a huge awful black monster came up and hit me straight on in the chest, knocking my breath out so that I could hardly breathe. I held the phone in my hand, but my mind was numb and my ears were barely hearing.

The doctor calmly went on talking, telling me that my lump was an infiltrating invasive lobular carcinoma, a specific medical term for breast Cancer. His words passed through my ears and my brain as if they were pebbles being thrown into a lake. The little rocks immediately disappeared below the water, leaving only a few surface ripples that went on and on through my mind. I didn't really hear the words that came across that phone line from my doctor that evening, but I felt the effects of the ripples. The ripples from those words changed my life forever. This happened to me on Tuesday, July 15, 2003.

My husband, Paul, and I had been eating our evening meal when the phone rang. The sun was still shining brightly outside, and it was warm. Seven days ago I had undergone a lumpectomy on my right breast. We had been anxiously awaiting the results of the pathology report from this surgery, but because my surgeon had explained before the surgery that 85 percent of these lumpectomies came back benign, I hadn't been mesmerized by this worry. I had continued on as if life were "normal." My breast was sore from the recent lumpectomy and was all bandaged up, but things were going well in my life. I really hadn't expected this kind of a diagnosis. After all, someone else always has Cancer, not me. This evening was the beginning of the unplanned journey for me. It was final and undeniable. I had Cancer.

Chapter 1

FACING THE WORST MAKES THE PROBLEM SEEM SMALLER

General Facts about Me

As a sixty-year-old happily married lady, I had the world by the tail that year of 2003. My second husband, Paul Dittmer, and I had been happily married for seventeen years. We shared seven children (six boys and one girl) between us. We had at that time fourteen beautiful and lively grandchildren. We were both retired and lived our lives in two places. We had a home in Grapevine, Texas, where we spent most of the spring, the fall, and part of the winter. We also enjoyed a home in Durango, Colorado, where we spent our summers and about two months of the winter. We were comfortable financially. I thought that we were in the best of all times.

I had always been careful to take care of myself. I had exercised regularly all of my life. I always saw a doctor when I got seriously sick and always had a yearly checkup and mammogram. I had always gotten regular mammograms each year for about twenty years. Most of those tests had been conducted at the Baylor Hospital in Grapevine, Texas. In December 2002, I had gone to see my doctor, a family practice doctor, to have my yearly physical exam and my mammogram. Everything in my life seemed to be normal. I felt secure since I was following all of the recommended guidelines. I felt that I was safe from devastating illnesses like Cancer.

I did monthly self-breast exams most months on my birthday anniversary (December 4), that is, January 4, February 4, March 4, etc. However, because we were busy traveling and getting ready to move back up to Colorado, I think that I missed doing my self-breast exams in April and May. I took care of my body and expected it to hold up healthily for many years.

Our life had been proceeding normally and was following my plans. I was always working on achieving my goals. Our leaving that spring from Texas had been difficult, however. Paul and I just couldn't seem to get all of our work and visiting completed. I wanted to leave, but I wanted our exit to be organized and complete. We finally left and arrived in Durango to find a landscape of wonderful beauty.

The winter had brought snows again, and the melt-off from these snows filled the rivers and the creeks and quenched the thirst of our droughty trees, brushes, and grasses. Colorado was marvelously alive that spring.

The Summer Devastation of 2002

In the summer of 2002, in Durango, we had lived through the horrible Mission Ridge wildfire. It burned 75,000 acres over a period of seven weeks. That summer had been terribly dry and destructive. Durango had been a place of fear because of the huge fire that devoured homes and all the forests just east of town. Our small, normally quiet city was a place of wild activity because the town was filled with over five hundred fire fighters who camped within our midst and were a constant reminder of the danger that licked at our door. It was scary to live in Durango during the summer of 2002. We were constantly afraid that fire would break out and might devour our home. The summer of 2002 was something that I had never experienced before. I had grown up in West Texas in the desert. Destructive forest or even grass fires were nonexistent in the world I lived in as a child.

When we arrived that spring in late May 2003, we found cool waters and new green growth had made the forests and the lands come back to life. This new life was a welcome sign of hope that made me feel renewed and positive that good things were in store for us and the land that year. I felt from the new environment that I saw that it was going to be an exciting year. That June, when I was filled with optimism and promises of renewal, I had no real idea of what lay ahead for me after the doctor called to tell me that I had Cancer. I had survived the devastation, the fears, and the ravages of the fires of 2002 in Durango, Colorado. Could I survive the devastations, the fears, and the ravages of the Cancer that I had to face? I wasn't sure.

But early that summer when we arrived (before I found "the lump"), we drove into our driveway to find that our yard was full of stirring, tall, growing green grass that was about a foot high with yellow flowers interspersed everywhere. The heads of the yellow dandelions, a weed, brightened the almost-solid carpet of green. The last time that we had seen our Colorado yard, it had been full of patches of snow, bare ground, and dead grass stubble left from the horrific summer of 2002, when we had *no* rain. Now all of our big Ponderosa pines looked alive and hearty, and even our new shrubs seemed to have survived the harshness of the drought of 2002 and would be healthy as they grew. Our yard was a cornucopia of wild grasses and flowers. What a sight!

We had a big job of unpacking and getting settled again into our Colorado house, but we accomplished this housekeeping job fairly quickly. We were able to go into town the next day after our arrival to get a few groceries and to wash and to clean up the truck that we had driven from Texas. It was easy this time to move immediately into the fun activities of Durango.

BREAST CANCER: THE UNPLANNED JOURNEY - LESSONS LEARNED

A Typical Week in My Life (Before I Knew I Had Cancer)

Durango Activities

Our activities that first week in Durango included seeing the Iron Horse Bicycle Rally, attending our church service, exercising three times in water aerobics classes, making a trip with friends to Bloomfield, New Mexico, going on two mountain/forest hikes, enjoying white-water rafting, making plans to host my high school reunion in Durango, and traveling to participate in a weekend camping trip on the Colorado/Utah border at the Dinosaur National Monument. I was physically active and very much enjoyed my adventures with other people. I thrived on exciting times and always pushed the limits just a bit. I had never planned on being sick and having Cancer take over my life.

The Iron Horse Bike Rally is an annual event in Durango. Bike riders come from all over the country to make the grueling ride up the mountain to Silverton in all kinds of weather. The bikers raced the Durango/Silverton Train on Saturday morning that year in nice sunny weather. Silverton is fifty-five miles up the mountains from Durango. I am always amazed that the riders are strong enough to complete this ride, much less race to do it. The altitude in Durango is 6,400 feet, and Silverton sits on the mountains at 11,050 feet. These riders face enormous battles of physical endurance in completing the ride. I stood and watched with great admiration for these riders who were tough enough. I thought that I would never be strong enough to finish such a match, but I didn't know what faced me ahead as I fought Cancer.

It was great to be greeted and welcomed home by our Colorado church family at Christ the King Lutheran Church. We immediately began again our routine of daily exercising by attending water aerobics with our exercise friends, the Mermaids. I exercised and talked with these friends, catching up on all of the news of the group. After our class that day, we attended a luncheon honoring the "Mermaids" with birthdays in May. I have many very close friends in this group of ladies. Even though I had been gone for several months, I was welcomed back immediately and was invited to participate in this celebration luncheon, even though I hadn't prepared a dish to share. These friends would prove to be invaluable to me during the year ahead when I fought my Cancer.

In my working to get into Colorado shape and to be as strong physically as the outdoorsy people in this town were, I immediately went on one of the hikes organized by the Seniors Outdoors Club of Durango. We hiked to the top of Animas Mountain (7,800 feet). I greatly admired the strength and the stamina of the "old" people in this club. Later that week, we went for a birding hike from Haviland Lake to Forebay Lake. This was fun and took less stamina because we didn't climb a mountain. This is a very unique and neat club in Durango. You must be over fifty-five to join, and most of the members are in their sixties and seventies. Many of them hiked and climbed the 14,000-feet-high mountains in Colorado.

I had set my goal for that summer to be able to hike and to climb some of these mountains myself. Because I lived most of the year at sea level, I found it very hard to keep up at these altitudes. I had trouble getting enough oxygen into my lungs and huffed and puffed a lot. This condition was embarrassing for me, but I was determined to do the necessary work so that I could get into Colorado shape. I did step aerobics five days a week in Texas, but somehow I was never strong enough when we got to Colorado. I believed that this was the summer that I would achieve my goal. Little did I know what the summer had in store for me.

White-Water Rafting

Paul and I decided that we needed to take advantage of the massive amounts of water that were crashing down the Animas River at this time, so we went white-water rafting. The trip was extraordinary. The river was flowing at the rate of 4,250 cubic feet of water per second. The Animas River was higher than it had been in three years, reducing the usual two-hour-long rafting trip to forty-five minutes. However, those forty-five minutes were packed with exciting waves, water holes, and rapids. We passed under many street and walking bridges, and the clearance under most of them was only about five feet. Because the river was so high, our guide could reach up with his hand and touch the bridges. The water in the river last year (2002) had barely trickled by in the very bottom of the riverbed. This day, the entire waterway was full of raging torrents. The river licked and pulled at everything along its sides. The normally visible rocks in the water were all covered. White-water waves were the only indications that the rocks that were so prominent in the river last summer were still there below.

White-water rafting has always been fun and exciting for me. I like the fast-moving pace of things and the slight fear that danger is just a little distance away. That afternoon, we paid our money and jumped aboard the old school bus to make the short trip to the entry point for the rafts on the Animas River. The wet suits that we donned were stinky and cold, but the tightly strapped life jackets helped me feel safe. The life jackets were built with straps on them behind one's head that were designed so that someone in the boat could grab onto this strap in order to pull a fellow passenger out of the river if the need arose. Since I had rafted in Panama and had seen rafts turn over in the rapids, I wanted to be well prepared to get out of this river and its cold water.

It was both exciting and fun to listen and to learn how to row and to follow the commands of the guide as four strangers learned to row as a team so that we could successfully navigate the difficult sections of this monstrous river. I enjoyed the fast and tough actions required to navigate through the treacherous rapids. I enjoyed the thought of the danger that would arise if I were thrown into the 37 degree Fahrenheit rushing water. However, our guide was skilled, and our raft made it through without tipping over. Several times, however, everyone clung to the raft in sheer desperation as the boat stood on end and then on its sides as it bounced through the rough waters. Often we couldn't tell which way we were even going because the water would spray over the boat, completely covering everything with dark, cold river water.

My heart raced, my muscles tensed, and the adrenalin flowed as we rounded the curve in the river where the difficult class III rapids were just ahead. Rapids in Colorado are usually rated as to their difficulty. A class I set of rapids contains rapids that are fairly easily negotiated. A class V set of rapids is very hard to raft through and very dangerous. The river boiled and raged continuously as we raced downstream. One of the young men in our boat was thrown into the frigid water just as we got though the class III rapids. Paul, my husband, stretched out over the water while holding onto the raft with one arm, reached with his other arm, and grabbed onto to the strap on the man's life jacket, and with extra strength that he got in this emergency that gave him super human powers, he pulled the man back into the safety of the raft. The young man was very wet and cold, but he would live to tell an exciting tale. Four strangers had worked together in the crisis situation.

We returned after our white-water rafting experience cold and exhilarated in the late afternoon. We had ridden the Lower Animas during the peak of its spring runoff! What an adventure! We had rafted through class III rapids! I loved physical excitement! I loved to be a part of the activity in the world around me! Little did I know that I would do nothing like this again for a whole year.

Friends

One afternoon, we met our friends, Marge and Bill Rebovich, and made a short trip to Bloomfield, New Mexico (about fifty miles away). We looked at some Indian artifacts (that were not as they had been advertised) and shopped at Sam's Discount Club. We enjoyed the visit and the time that we spent together. I always found that when you are driving, you could have some very good uninterrupted talking time. We had many good friends in Colorado and very much enjoyed the camaraderie that we shared with them. Our friends made our life richer. *Friends would turn out to be very valuable resources for encouragement and strength when I battled Cancer.*

I was also busy getting ready to host my McCamey (Texas) High School Class reunion on July 25, 26, and 27. Paul helped me get everything together, and we carefully made the plans. It looked like we were going to have a fairly good turnout. Everyone seemed to be excited about coming to Durango. One of my classmates was coming all the way from Turkey. It promised to be a busy and fun summer.

Family

One of the reasons that I really felt at home in Colorado was that I had family that lived nearby. Nearly all of my children and relatives lived in Texas. However, my cousin, Connie, and her husband, Bill Twilley, lived in Farmington, New Mexico, about sixty miles away. They came up to share a Sunday dinner and afternoon with us that week. This physical closeness allowed us to visit often and gave me a nice "family" feeling. We especially enjoyed our time together that Sunday afternoon. It was our first visit that summer. I didn't realize that because of the activities related to my Cancer treatments, we wouldn't see each other again that year.

Last Outing Before Cancer

Thursday afternoon, June 5, we packed to go on a three-day campout to Dinosaur National Monument. Hurriedly we finished our work and loaded our four-wheel-drive car with our tent, sleeping bags, and other supplies. We were finally ready for our first camping trip in Colorado, and I was both excited and apprehensive!

At eight the next morning, we met other members of the San Juan Basin Archaeology Society in Durango. The drive to Dinosaur National Park was over a three-hundred-mile all-day trip. The trip took us north and west all day. We nearly ran into a deer trying to cross the busy highway outside of Ouray. We met up with our group again at Fruta, just outside of Grand Junction, and drove on through the desert to the tiny town of Jensen. Jensen was about ten miles from the park entrance.

We reached the park at about 5:00 p.m. and went to the campground. The beautiful campground sat right beside the Green River (famed for the summer Mountain Men Rendezvous in the 1830s). The Mountain Men were the brave, independent trappers who worked in the Western mountains before the settlers came. We all chose our camping sites and started to set up camp. The evening was lovely. Paul and I managed to get our tent up without too much trouble. After this successful feat, I had hopes that this camping trip might work out to be okay after all. This was the very first time that Paul and I had camped.

Although the overall environment was lovely, with the blue river running through the camp and the nearby mountains providing a dramatic backdrop, the campsites were dirty and dusty. Nothing I could do seemed to settle the dust, and I decided that I had just better get accustomed to it. Fortunately, I was able to keep our tent very clean and therefore had a small space that I felt comfortable in. It was really nice to get into our tent in the early evenings, to take off my clothes after having taken a sponge bath at the restroom, to wash my feet, and to feel clean in my own special area. I curled up in my sleeping bag and, with my flashlight/lamp, was able to enjoy a bit of reading in the wild. The birds and the campground evening sounds were very pleasant and peaceful.

We spent the weekend driving around the area and climbing up the mountainsides so that we could view the many ancient Indian petroglyphs in the area. We saw the dinosaur bones that are so well preserved in the rocks at Dinosaur National Monument. We enjoyed lots of good campfire talks with our friends and eating food cooked outside. It was an exciting three days.

This first-time experience of camping, for me, had been successful. I had managed to sleep on my cot in my sleeping bag, although the nights got very cold. I had learned to live with the constant smell of mosquito repellant. I had managed with a bathroom that was 200 yards from my bed at night. I hadn't starved on camping food and had really enjoyed the hikes and the outings that we had taken. The friendly chipmunks had been an entertainment at our campsite. I decided that we could now camp in Colorado. Since the outdoors is such a part of life in Colorado, I thought that Paul and I had climbed up a rung on the ladder toward the goal of our becoming real Coloradans.

When we got back home on Monday, June 9, we unpacked and I really enjoyed a long shower. There had been no showers in our camp so I had gone the entire four days with only "washrag baths." It was really nice to be home. We had enjoyed a wonderful week, and I now expected the rest of the summer to follow in the same manner. Our lives were very busy with lots of fun activities and good friends. Life was good! I never imagined how things could change so quickly.

Finding "the Lump"

Self-Breast Exam that Was Different

On Tuesday evening, June 10, after a day of working as a volunteer at the Humane Society Thrift Store, I had casually begun to perform my self-breast exam in bed. I tried to do one of these exams at the beginning of each month. I knew that my doctors and mammography techs always told me to do it each month on my birthday anniversary, the fourth, but I often forgot to do it on that exact day. Sometimes I had even forgotten it for the entire month. I had never felt that I actually knew what I was feeling for. My breasts were full of lumps. How could I possibly find a new one? I just went through the motions so that when I was asked I could honestly say that I did self-breast examinations.

That night, I lay in bed and raised my left arm to begin the breast exam. Everything felt like it always did—very lumpy. When I switched hands and my left hand examined my right breast, I felt a very hard nodule under the right nipple. This knot felt *very* different. I put my right arm down and felt of my left breast again to see if I could find anything there that felt like what I had felt on the right side. My left breast felt soft and flexible, altogether different from what I had felt on my right side. I felt again my right breast because surely I had just made a mistake. Again, I quickly felt the very large peanut just under my nipple. I checked my left breast again and then my right. Each time, I felt the same thing. I collected my courage and whispered to Paul that I had found a lump in my right breast.

We had been watching television, and he immediately turned the set off. He came over to the bed and quietly sat down on his side. I asked him if he wanted to feel it. He said that he was sure that he couldn't feel it and tried to encourage me by saying that most lumps were benign and harmless. He said that we would have to get to a doctor to get it checked out. He lay down beside me, and we turned off the lights.

It was a long night for me. I thought and thought and thought. I am strong and *very* healthy. How could I have a lump in my breast? What was this dark thing that had grown in my body? Should I immediately stop my estrogen patch? How long would I live if this were Cancer? God, what was I going to do?

Sandy's Breast Cancer

My breast self-examination and the lump reminded me of one of my Colorado friends, Sandy. The first time that we had attended Christ the King Lutheran Church in Durango in the summer of 2000, there was a nice-looking tall lady named Sandy, who had no hair on her head. She was entirely bald. However, she was happy and seemed strong. I talked to her and discovered that she had breast Cancer and had lost her hair from the chemotherapy that she had undergone. She said that she didn't want to wear a wig. She proudly walked around bald as if it were a badge of honor. It certainly was a badge of courage. I was impressed with her strength and bravery from the very beginning.

Over these last two years, I had watched Sandy's hair grow back. She had continued to be an active member of our church. One of her children had a baby, and she became a grandmother. Life seemed to be going well for her when I had left Colorado in March 2003. However, when we returned this summer and I saw her the week before, I found that her Cancer had come back and had spread to her lungs. She was now fighting to live. Her immune system was so low that no one could visit her. Because I was her friend, I got regular e-mails on her condition. I always wanted to keep up with how this courageous lady was doing. From the last reports, it didn't sound like she was doing well. I was afraid that she would die soon from breast Cancer that had spread to her lungs. Her possible death really scared me since it looked like I might face the same battle.

Learning to Live with "the Lump"

Living One Day at a Time

With much difficulty and "what if" thinking, I made it through that first night. The next day, Wednesday, June 12, 2003, Paul and I went about our regular activities. We didn't talk about the lump, except that I told Paul that I would wait a day to see if the lump might disappear. I hoped that I had just made a mistake. We went on the Wednesday Wanderers hike with the Seniors Outdoors around Durango West II. The outside bright sunshine and fresh air helped to immediately lift my spirits. I hiked and talked. I told one of my good friends, who had been a nurse, that I had found a lump. She immediately recommended her nurse practitioner as someone that I should see. She was encouraging, and I told her that I would get an appointment as soon as I could. It was a big step for me to open up enough to tell a friend about the lump. By talking about it, I was making it a reality.

That evening, my friend and her husband came to our house for dinner. It was a nice evening, and the lump was not in the forefront of my mind. After our company left and the kitchen was cleaned, I went up to bed to do another exam. After only a few seconds, I found the lump just as hard as it had been the night before. I had not made a mistake.

I knew now that I had to begin the frustrating search to find out if the lump that I had was Cancer or not. I wanted an immediate diagnosis, but I couldn't get one. I couldn't just call up my doctor and get an appointment. The doctor's clinic that we had been using had closed, and I didn't really even have a general practitioner in Durango.

Thursday morning, we went to water aerobics as usual. My good friend, Marge, who was a retired nurse from Mercy Hospital in Durango, attended this class. I immediately cornered her and, while we were exercising, told her about finding the lump. She asked me questions about it. She recommended that I see her doctor and then proceeded to tell me about a time a few years ago when she found a hard lump in her breast that felt like a small piece of gravel. She waited three weeks before she went to the doctor. The surgeon she went to could not feel her lump and told her to wait a while longer. She waited three more weeks and then went back to the surgeon and told him to take the lump out. It was worrying her, and she wanted it out. The surgeon took it out in a simple day operation, and it was benign. Everything was fine. The surgeon told her not to fiddle with her breasts so much. We both laughed, and I felt a little better.

Accepting the Worst

Because I was feeling more worried by the minute, I decided that I had to come to grips with this thing, this possible Cancer seed that I had found. I could not live in fear all of the time and be happy and productive, so I used my old psychological training. What was the worst thing that could come of this? I thought again logically. I had done what I thought that I should have done. I had examined my breasts nearly every month. I had done my last exam recently, and the lump had not been there, so it had not been growing very long. I had had a mammogram in December of 2002. The lump wasn't present then. The lump could only have been growing for a short while. If it was cancer, the doctors would recommend that I have a mastectomy. They would take off my breast. That couldn't be too bad. I reasoned that I was old enough now that being a beauty queen or a sex object was not my thing anyway. I had talked it over with Paul, and he assured me that he would love me even if I were flat-chested. So if the worst thing happened, the lump turned out to be Cancer, and the doctors would remove my breast, I decided that I could live with that. If I accepted the worst-case scenario, maybe I wouldn't feel so bad.

I had a good friend in my water aerobics class who had undergone a double mastectomy many years ago, and she was old now and was happy and useful. I was not too concerned about how I looked anymore. I decided that my breasts had nothing to do with my self-esteem or my femaleness. Paul would love me the same with or without my right breast. So after *I faced the worst possible outcome, the problem didn't quite seem so big*. I slept better that night.

Friday, I exercised at the Recreation Center with my friend, Therese. She was participating in a big Cancer Walk that Friday evening. We exercised together and talked a lot. I told Therese about finding the lump. She was immediately concerned and told me that one of her sisters had died of breast Cancer. She recommended that I see her doctor and encouraged me to get in to see her right away. I went home and began making calls to several doctors' offices. Most of the recommended doctors were not seeing any new patients. I explained that I was a close friend of Nurse Marge Rebovich and that I had found a lump in my breast. However, nothing helped. I gave up on getting in to see a doctor and called the highly recommended nurse practitioner and was able to get an appointment five days later. I would have liked to have gotten in sooner, but I was making peace with my demon, the lump, so I thought that I would be able to stand to wait. I was happy to at least have a date to see a medical person about this new condition.

That Sunday evening, I called my mother, my sister, and my daughter and told them about the lump. Mary Joy, my daughter, was an ob-gyn doctor who was finishing her last year of residency in a suburb in Detroit, Michigan. She instructed me not to leave the doctor's office next week without a prescription for a mammogram or a sonogram. Since I had already faced what I thought was the worst scenario, I was able to talk about the lump without getting all emotional and crying. I was thankful for that small ability.

Chapter 2

EVERYTHING MOVES SO SLOWLY

Diagnosing

First Appointment with Nurse Practitioner

Finally, Wednesday, June 18, arrived, and I went in to see the Nurse Practitioner who had been recommended to me. She was very kind, efficient, and thorough. She too could easily feel the lump. She prescribed a mammogram and a sonogram and hinted that we would probably have a surgeon look at it even if the mammogram and the sonogram came back okay. She must have called and gotten me special considerations in the radiology department because I was able to leave her office and go directly down to get my mammogram. After the mammogram, the technician stayed late in order to give me the radiologist's report. I received very special and immediate attention at this phase of my diagnosis. I wish that it could all have gone so efficiently.

Mammogram

A mammogram is an x-ray picture of one's breast. Women hate to undergo a mammogram because they squeeze and mash your breast in the process of taking the picture. Mammograms are uncomfortable, and some women would say that they actually hurt. However, mammograms are critical in the diagnosis of most breast Cancers, so I have always gotten an annual mammogram for the last twenty years. It was not busy that late afternoon in the lab, and the mammogram tech was very kind and concerned about me. She took me back immediately to do the mammogram. She could feel the lump in my right breast.

After the completion of the test, she got the radiologists to look at the film and informed me that it was definitely *not* the raging kind of Cancer but that they just didn't know for sure what it was. They needed to see my last mammogram that, of course, was in Texas. Upon hearing that the lump was not the raging kind of Cancer, I felt a little better as I left the hospital that afternoon. I didn't really know what the raging kind of Cancer was, but I was glad that I didn't have it. I needed any little glimmer of hope that I could get at this time. I now had an active job to do to get my mammograms sent from Texas.

I am an active kind of person. I enjoyed doing things. Activity kept me from thinking horrible thoughts about the lump. After this progress in my efforts to get a diagnosis, Paul and I talked about our immediate plans. Everyone in Durango seemed caring and competent. At this time, I decided to run this medical adventure here in Durango rather than to go immediately back to Texas. This decision very much affected the way that my Cancer treatment went. However, at the time and with the limited knowledge that we had, this seemed to be a good decision.

The mammography technician called up the imaging department and got me an appointment for my sonogram. Unfortunately, I couldn't get this appointment until six days later. I had more waiting to endure.

Passing the Time Waiting

I nervously waited for the days to pass. I had nightmares at night. I thought that I had Cancer, but I didn't say it to anyone. I was too afraid that if I said the "*C*" word, it might come true. I worried quietly and alone. Paul felt sure that it was just a fibrous lump that was not malignant. I was hoping that the sonogram would show this lump to be just a cyst, something that we would leave alone and not worry about.

I started reading some breast Cancer literature. I talked about finding the lump with my friends. I was amazed to find out how many of them had gone through similar scares. They all told me their stories. One lady that I worked with at the Thrift Store told me that she had Cancer and had undergone a mastectomy. She never told anyone outside of her immediate family about the Cancer before but felt like she should tell me about it so that I would know that you could be "okay" after having had breast Cancer. I thought that she was very kind.

One friend of mine said that she had lumps that appeared all of the time. Her lumps didn't show up on a mammogram or on a sonogram. Each time she finds one of these new lumps, she goes directly to a surgeon here in town who drains each lump to make sure that it isn't Cancer, and she goes on with her life.

I never knew so many women had these problems before. Anyway, I was attempting to get better educated in this area, and I was praying. It was difficult waiting. I kept as busy as I could. I tried not to think about the lump, but it always weighed heavy on my back. On the outside, our lives appeared to be moving along as if nothing were wrong. However, I carried a huge pack of worries every minute of every day and night that I could never put down. I was beginning to learn a very important lesson in this battle (the unplanned journey)—*nothing moved as quickly as I would have liked.* My life was filled all along the way with many of hours of waiting.

Sonogram

A sonogram is a picture that is taken of a part of the body using sound waves. Doctors use sonograms to check on the development and the sex of babies in the early months of pregnancy. Sonograms are easy and do not hurt. A technician uses what looks like a microphone and rolls or rubs it across your body. A machine that is attached by a cord to the microphone unit somehow draws the picture of the inside of your body below the "microphone unit."

Finally, my appointment for the sonogram, June 24, arrived, and I went to the hospital. Having a sonogram is as "easy as pie." Again, the technician could feel the lump. She took pictures of the breast and went to consult the radiologist. He immediately came in and ran the sonogram himself, felt the lump, and told me that they didn't know what it was. He said that it needed to be taken out.

Surgeon's Appointment

I left the hospital and drove home. The lump was not a cyst. Everyone that I had gone to could feel it. By now, I had just about given up on it magically going away. When I arrived home, I called the surgeons who had been recommended to me to get an appointment. I couldn't get in with my first-choice surgeon, Dr. Dwight Dover, until July 28. This was over a month away. I surely didn't want to wait this long to find out what this awful thing was in my body. The only thing that I could do to maybe speed things up was to get on his standby list in case someone canceled. My good friend, Marge Rebovich, told me that she would talk to Dr. Dover and see what she could do to get me in earlier. Fortunately, the scheduler for Dr. Dover called in the next couple of days and said that I could get in at 3:00 p.m. on Wednesday, July 2. I happily took the appointment.

We had planned to leave for a visit in Texas that Wednesday morning, but we delayed our departure. Getting this problem diagnosed was number one on the importance ladder at this time. Not knowing what this thing was caused me to live in a strange dark hole. The only way out of the hole was to find out what the lump was. I felt the foreign matter nightly, hoping against hope that it would just disappear. I couldn't tell if it was growing. I couldn't leave it alone long enough to notice any change. It remained very hard.

Accepting My Condition

While I waited to see the surgeon, I reached deep into my soul for some brightness, and I never lost all hope. It was really scary, however. I had experienced many glorious mountaintops since my marriage to Paul in 1986. I guessed that I was due some "hard times," and the lump was certainly throwing my life and emotions into a downward spiraling spin. I did not know what was ahead, but I knew that there was a plan and that I would be all right in that plan. Our life went on, but Paul and I both recognized that I was in this deep hole awaiting the light that would drive the monster away. The lumpectomy or biopsy should be a "walk in the park" compared to the nightmare that I was living in, not knowing whether I had Cancer or not.

I still did everything I always did, and I hoped that soon this whole thing would be over. Hopefully, I would feel like a silly goose for having worried so. Now that I had a doctor's appointment, I felt sure that the lump would surely just disappear. I remembered how when you take your car with the bad engine noise to the shop that the noise in the engine magically disappears when the mechanic shows up to fix it. What if I had gotten everyone upset and the lump turned out to be nothing? I would be very embarrassed.

However, each night, when I lay down in my bed, I felt the lump again. It didn't go away. I faced some very difficult nights. When I wasn't busy and working, I could think of all the things that might happen if the lump turned out to be Cancer. I thought and worried and thought some more. I stayed awake. One night, when I couldn't sleep between 11:00 p.m. and 4:00 a.m., I finally resorted to sitting down at my computer and writing about my worries and my feelings as follows:

> It is one thirty in the morning. The house is dark and quiet. Mr. Boots (my cat) and I are the only ones who are awake in this world. It is pitch dark outside. There is no moon. None of my neighbors are awake. I am absolutely alone with my thoughts and "THE LUMP."

I now realized that what I had written that late night described quite well the darkness and the aloneness that I felt when I lay down in my bed each night to try to sleep. It was a very black and difficult time for me. I couldn't figure out how this could be happening to me. I was strong and healthy. What could have gone wrong in my body? What had I done to have caused this? Why was God allowing this to happen to me?

In the daytimes, we went on with our lives. I went to water aerobics, met with my Stephens Ministry caregiver's group, went on hikes with the Seniors Outdoors Club, hosted a potluck, entertained our friends, and worked at the Humane Society Thrift Store. However, everywhere I went, I knew that I had something extra to carry—the knowledge that I had the lump in my breast that might be something awful. I didn't think about it in the daytime, but at night, a specter would haunt me. However, it was my specter, my lump, and no one could face it but me. So I did.

Chapter 3

MAKE THE JOURNEY ONE STEP AT A TIME

Meeting My Surgeon

I began to realize about this time that I really was trying to rid myself of what I was afraid was a horrible monster by taking very small steps. There was no way that I could just wiggle my nose like Samantha did in *Bewitched*, the old-time TV show, and get rid of the lump. I had to do one simple thing at time. I had to follow the path that seemed to be laid out for me. My steps after finding the lump so far had been to tell everyone about the lump, to find a doctor and to make an appointment, to follow the nurse practitioner's orders to get the mammogram and the sonogram, to keep following orders, and to obtain an appointment with my surgeon. I was moving down the road one small step at a time. This was not the road that I had chosen or wanted to be on, but it was what was assigned to me.

It was July 2, and I had started on the unplanned journey a little less than a month ago when I had found the lump. To me, it seemed like it had taken a very long time to come this far. On July 2, we went to town and met with my surgeon, Dr. Dover. His reputation in Durango placed him as the best surgeon in our area. He was very nice, caring, and knowledgeable. He easily felt the lump, finding it without my help. He said that I had two options. Number 1, he could do a needle biopsy, but this method was only 90 percent accurate. Number 2, he could take the lump out, which would allow the lab to do a completely accurate diagnosis of whether it was benign or not. If the needle biopsy came back bad, then he would have to go in and take out the lump anyway. So I opted to have him take the lump out the first time. This way, I would know for sure what it was.

He could do the surgery on Friday, July 11, at 11:00 a.m. I was ready. He did give me some information that greatly relieved my mind. He said that 85 percent of the lumps that were taken out in the United States were benign. I really liked odds of that sort. I slept better that night, knowing that the unplanned journey (hopefully) would end on July 11. I hoped that I would know when I got the pathology report from the lab that this horrible time had ended positively. I thought that I could all of a sudden see the light at the end of the tunnel. There was surely hope that this had been a false alarm. I now had the job of living my life while I waited again.

Passing the Time

Off to Texas

We left Durango on Thursday, July 3, the day after I talked to the surgeon, to go to Texas to my family reunion that was to be held on Saturday, July 5. I always enjoyed seeing all of my family. My mother was ninety that summer and was in excellent health. I visited with my cousins, nieces, nephews, children, grandchildren, and miscellaneous relatives. It was wonderful renewing family ties. I didn't tell anyone that I might have Cancer. This family gathering was a very pleasant distracting interlude on my road to determine if the lump was Cancer.

Back to Durango with Two Grandchildren

When we left Texas, we brought two of our grandchildren, Colten (nine) and Lilli (six), with us for a visit. The trip back was a long 800 miles that we drove in two days. The children were wonderful all along the way. I taught Colten how to read the map and the road signs so he always knew where we were. It kept him from asking a hundred times the old familiar trip question, "When are we going to be there?" I didn't have time to think about the lump while caring for these fabulous and active children. When we reached Durango, it was a busy time as we took the kids around to see some of the sites.

On Wednesday, July 9, we took the grandchildren with us to the surgeon's office for my pre-op appointment. Fortunately, they were very good children, and we left them sitting in the waiting room while we talked to Dr. Dover. Lilli and Colten went with us wherever we went during this time of preparation, even for the prehospital tests and check-in. I took books and colors with us so they had something to do while they waited. They were wonderful and seemed to understand that Grandmother had to do these things. They were my most loving supporters during this time and never allowed me to feel sorry for myself. It was great to have this wonderful distraction as I walked on the unplanned journey.

The Lumpectomy

On Friday, July 11, the scheduled day of my surgery, we still had Lilli and Colten with us. Since the surgeon had assured me that the odds were 85 percent that the lump was benign, I wasn't afraid. Lilli's and Colten's father, our sixth son, Paul Damian Hyde, and his wife, Stephanie, were flying in that day. I was so confident about the surgery that I told Paul to just take me to the hospital and leave me and go on to the airport with Lilli and Colten so that he could pick up Paul Damian and Stephanie. I assured him that I would be all right until he could get back to pick me up about 4:00 p.m. I was being very brave. I was not going to fall to pieces and cause too much of a burden for other people with this little simple surgery.

When Paul left me that morning, my good friend, Marge Rebovich, arrived to stay with me. It was quite a surprise and a big blessing to see her. She was a perfect companion because she was a nurse and knew so much about what was happening. She stayed with me through the entire procedure. How lucky could I have been? Even though I had told Paul not to worry that I really wasn't scared at all, I was. It was so comforting to have the confidence and the knowledge of my good friend to bolster my spirits. *Please be there in person for your friends who go through similar experiences even if they tell you that they don't need you.* I really needed a loved one's presence. Marge with her vast experience knew that I needed someone and filled my needs completely. I will forever be grateful for her special kindness.

Shortly after Marge arrived, I went into the preoperation area, got undressed, and lay down on a bed (stretcher). The doctor came in and checked me. The nurse started an IV and gave me some medicine to help me relax. I left Marge and was wheeled into the surgery room. They draped a sheet like a curtain over my chest just below my chin so that I could not see what they were doing to my breast. A nurse anesthesiologist sat down near my head. She explained that she would stay with me all of the time. She held my hand and often patted my head. Her presence and calm voice was comforting and reassuring to me throughout the entire operation. The doctor and the nurses went to work. I didn't really feel any pain. The first few numbing shots were painful, but then I didn't really feel anything else in my breast area.

Dr. Dover talked and dictated technical notes for the nurse to write down about the surgery. He also gave her parts and pieces of the lump. I just lay there. The nurse anesthesiologist stayed with me all of the time and constantly reassured me that everything was going well. It was over in just a few minutes (not more than thirty minutes). When everything was done, Dr. Dover came from the other side of the curtain that was hanging over my chest and told me that the surgery had gone well. I, of course, asked him if he thought that the lump was Cancer. He would not answer this question but assured me that in a few days, he would get the pathology report from the lab and then I would know whether it was Cancer or not. I just knew that the lump was gone, and for the moment, everything was fine.

A nurse wheeled me into the recovery room where I dozed for a while. Marge was waiting for me. Soon another nurse came and suggested that it was time for me to sit up in a kind of reclining chair, so I struggled to see if my muscles still worked. They did, and I was able to crawl out of bed into the reclining chair. There I drank some juice and ate a small package of cookies. I was feeling less groggy, and it wasn't long before Paul arrived.

After the Surgery

When I had gained full consciousness and mobility, I was wheeled to the front of the hospital, where Paul picked me up in our car. I felt pretty good. I gave Marge a big hug and a thank-you, and we said good-bye. On our way home, we stopped by the Recreation Center so that I could see Paul Damian and Stephanie. They had all gone swimming while Paul had come to the hospital to be with me. We went home immediately after I watched them swim a while, and I rested that evening. My breast was wrapped up tightly in tape. I had received instructions to wear a very tight bra and to keep this tape just like it was. I was sore, but the doctor had given me pain pills that helped to keep me comfortable.

Paul Dittmer and Paul Damian are both good cooks, so I didn't worry about doing any of the normal "hosting" jobs. The next day, I rode with Paul Damian and his family on the Durango/Silverton train. It was an all-day excursion, and I was really tired when we got home that evening. However, it had been a wonderful opportunity to spend some quality time with my son and his family. The constant bouncing and jostling of the train was a little difficult on my sore breast. I was very thankful that it was so tightly bandaged.

By Saturday evening, however, the tape had started causing my chest to itch and itch. I tried to scratch through the tape but was unsuccessful. I spent a miserable night Saturday and a bad day Sunday with a very itchy boob. I discovered that I am allergic to hospital tape. The tape breaks me out, causing an aggravating skin rash.

I very much enjoyed the visit with my son, Paul Damian. He and his family left on Monday afternoon, and I began helping with Vacation Bible School on Tuesday, July 15. I used work and activity to keep me from worrying about the pathology report that we were waiting for. I am not an especially good person when I have to wait. I could never have gotten through this part of my life if I had not been very busy.

Cancer for Sure

The Doctor Called

My surgeon called in the early evening of Tuesday, July 15, just before five. He told me that I had Cancer. The moment that I described in the first page of this book was very real. Dr. Dover told me to get a pencil so that I could write things down. I called for Paul to get on the phone with me, and the doctor proceeded to tell us the story.

From the pathology report, the lump was determined to be an infiltrating invasive lobular carcinoma. The surgeon did not get all of the Cancer in his cuttings this time. He did not get "clear margins" is what the pathology report said. The doctor proceeded to try to help us by giving us more facts. Out of one hundred breast Cancers, this kind of Cancer accounts for fifteen to twenty of them. This Cancer starts in the breast, where milk is produced (in the lobules).

He had cut out tissue in this lumpectomy that was over an inch in diameter, but the lab report showed that the tumor was too close to the edge of these cuttings in a couple of places. He did not get all of the Cancer. He also found lobular carcinoma in situ in my breast, which by itself is not normally removed. This is just a form of "Cancer" (I think) that they watch. However, since he was going to have to go back into my breast to be sure that he got all of the Cancer, he would remove this "Cancer" also.

In this second surgery, he would also do a sentinel node biopsy, which should tell us whether the invasive Cancer had spread anywhere else in my body. Apparently, the Cancer first spreads into other parts of the body through lymph nodes. The lymph nodes under the arms are the ones that usually get the traveling Cancer cells first. The sentinel nodes are the first ones to be affected. If the sentinel nodes are clear, the odds are that the Cancer is contained within the lump in the breast. If the lymph nodes were clear, he said that I would have to do radiation treatments, after which, I should be clear of any Cancer and would be okay.

Dr. Dover explained that we could meet again on Thursday morning, July 17, to go through the "if then" charts and to schedule the next surgery date. I wanted to have this next surgery as quickly as possible. I didn't want this Cancer to continue to grow in my body. He assured me that the Cancer was growing very slowly. He stated that it had been in my breast for several years.

When Paul and I hung up the phones, we just didn't quite know what to do. We hugged, and I continued to cry. Paul tried in his way to reassure me. He insisted that we would do whatever it took to fight this Cancer and to get it out of my body. I was lucky to have such wonderful support, even though at that moment, I didn't feel a bit lucky.

Telling My Family and Friends

A little while, after hanging up the phone with the doctor, I set about to call a couple of my dear Durango friends. Talking to a few others and telling them of my plight seemed to be the next steps to take on my journey, which had now turned fully into Cancer—the unplanned journey. I called Marge, my nurse friend, first. I wanted to talk to her right away. I next called my doctor daughter, Mary Joy (MJ), and got her answering machine. I left a message.

Mary Joy is our seventh child, our only girl, and is an ob-gyn doctor. Soon her husband, Tarl, who is also a doctor, called me back. He talked to me in his doctor's voice, and I told him what I had just heard from my surgeon here. He said that Mary Joy was on call nights this month and was at the hospital but that he would have her call me. Mary Joy called me back quickly. I cried and so did she. I had a loving conversation with her promising to look up things about my Cancer. She hated that she couldn't be here with me for what lay ahead. She is in her last year of residency in Detroit, Michigan. I assured her that there was nothing that she could do; that I had lots of loving, supportive friends to help me; and that everything would be all right. She is a fabulous daughter, and it helped me to talk to her, to know that she loves me so much, and that she would help me through this ordeal.

I called my mother and my sister, Karen, next. I called my son, John. I talked to John's wife, Shelley, also. They were all very loving and very concerned. I called my baby son, Paul Damian who had been visiting us when I had the lumpectomy. He told me reassuringly that he had seen lots of weaker people than me lick Cancer and that he was sure that I would overcome it also. He really wanted me to come back to Texas where I had family around. I promised him that I would return if I thought there was any need. Stephanie, Paul Damian's wife, immediately called me back to talk a few minutes. I called Cristi, the wife of our fourth son, and left a message. She called me back quickly also. I told her to deliver my Cancer news to her husband, James.

A little later that evening, Paul's Aunt Eunice from Wenatchee, Washington, called "out of the clear blue." She wanted to know the result of my biopsy. She and I were amazingly close. We were not related by blood at all, but I felt as close to her as if she were a very special aunt of mine. I did love her, and I think that she loved me. I hated to tell her my bad news, but I did. She had fought colon Cancer about fifteen years ago so she had more knowledge about what lay ahead for me than I did. Aunt Eunice died from metastasized colon Cancer in 2006, and I miss her today. At the time that I had Cancer, she was my special supporting friend.

Living the First Night with "the Monster"

When I had talked to the doctor on the phone that evening, I began my plunge into the deep depths of a dark hole. I had been clinging to the side of that dark hole, with my nose poking out just above the rim before I received this final Cancer news. I had been hoping desperately that everything was going to be all right. The doctor's call pushed me down, and I fell and fell and fell. I was so depressed that I could do nothing for the next twenty-four hours. I couldn't do anything but cry and feel the despair that I would compare in my desperate and dramatic moments to what Christ might have felt in the Garden of Gethsemane when he prayed, "Lord, let this cup pass from me, if it be Thy will." Jesus's pleading with his Father shows at some level the deep despair and fear that he felt that dire night when he knew what was in store for him at his capture and his crucifixion. It wasn't God's will that he be saved from His destiny, so Jesus died on the cross. There wasn't any way out of this sentence for me either. Please note that I am not implying that I am Christ-like or that this is a God-caused happening.

I finally went upstairs that fateful night and did my nightly bedtime chores. My mouth by now was full of ulcer sores from the stress that I had been undergoing daily in my worrying, so my nightly tooth brushing was painful. Doing my nightly chores and following my regular routine, however, was somehow comforting. I got into bed and cried some more. After a while of sleeplessness, I got out of bed and wrote in my diary the following words:

> I think that this thing will be all right in the end. I just hate to have to go through this. I know that we don't have a choice about what we do in life. We don't get to choose our paths. I do believe that God is in control, but I don't believe that God gives us

Cancer or even causes it to grow. I believe that because of the hormones that I have taken or because I lived in West Texas in the carcinogenic atmosphere of the oil field when I was growing up or because of some other fluke, the Cancer grew in my body. I do believe that God had the power to stop it, but I think that most of the time, he allows the laws of the earth to rule. I believe that he only steps in and alters the natural course of things occasionally. I do not know why God did not keep this from happening to me, but I know quite certainly that he will give me the strength and the courage and the support to see this thing through to the end. I will not walk this road alone (thank goodness).

As I lay in bed that night of the unplanned journey, I knew that I would grieve for a while. I decided that I was not going to leave this house until I was ready. I was going to work to nurture my body and my mind. I would have to learn to accept the presence of this Cancer, but for right now, I was still in shock. How could this happen to me? I now had to replan my entire set of goals for the summer. However, accepting the fact that I had Cancer was big. It took me several days to climb up this huge step on my road. I got to sleep late that night and slept fitfully.

Hibernating

My general reaction to the news that the lump was Cancer was to just stop doing everything. Nothing seemed important anymore. I had no desire to put up the dishes or to make the bed. None of this mattered to me. I did not go out. For about twenty-four hours, I cuddled in my cocoon. I talked to only the people that called me. I hibernated, cried, and tried to figure out what I was going to do. Paul carried the load of the cleaning and the cooking. After twenty-four hours of wallowing and doing nothing, I finally began to read and to study about my disease.

I have always believed in the power of the mind, and I had had premonitions that the lump was Cancer. I had dreamed very vividly on the previous Sunday night, July 13, before the doctor had called on Tuesday, July 15, telling me that the biopsy report showed that I had breast Cancer. The dream that I had experienced was very detailed and showed that part of the lump was serious Cancer, while the other part was not. My dream had been very real and lifelike. When I awoke after having experienced the dream, I felt terribly scared and almost sick. I didn't tell anyone about my dream. As it turned out, my dream had been completely right—it hadn't given me the technical names or details of the Cancer, but the overall picture seemed to have been almost perfect. Was my dream premonition, fear, or enlightenment? I thought that telling anyone or acknowledging this dream in any way before the actual diagnosis might have made it more likely to have come true, so I kept it bottled inside. Now that I knew that I had Cancer, I could tell the dream. My dreams often provided logs that were always feeding the fire of fear that I had burning within me.

Waiting to See the Surgeon Again

At this time I was devastated, and Paul was upset. The news that I had Cancer really left both of us reeling. This news was *not* what we had wanted. I was too healthy and too strong to have Cancer. I had never really been sick in my life before. What would we do? How could I accept this? Was I going to die? What in the world was God doing, allowing this to happen to me? No one in my immediate family, except my Grandmother Stacy, had ever had Cancer. I had nursed my children. I had started and stopped my menses at the normal time. I was not supposed to have Cancer. Whatever would we do?

As Paul and I attempted to come to grips with my diagnosis, we surfed the Web and read and read and read about breast Cancer. I had lots of questions to ask that I wrote down in my notebook. Knowledge was the only thing that Paul and I could find to arm ourselves against the fears of Cancer. We had to do something. Neither of us really knew very much about breast Cancer beyond the fact that people died from it. We had to somehow get our arms around the problem so that we would be able to decide what to do about it. I truly wished that I did not have to walk this particular road, but I didn't know what God's plan was for me. I somehow knew that I just had to continue walking. This was not what I had planned to do in the summer of 2003. I had not planned this journey. I was forced to reluctantly go on the unplanned journey.

Physically I was not really very comfortable, and I was still a little weak from the first lumpectomy. My right breast that had undergone the lumpectomy was itching terribly. It was hard to scratch the itch because of the incision, stitches, and the binding tape. Plus, if I touched the wound, the itchy place, very hard, it would hurt. What was I to do? My right breast was all yellowish from the bruising of the surgery and from where the doctor had injected the deadening shots. My right nipple was crooked. It looked down all of the time. My right "boob" was also now smaller than the left. The way my right breast looked, I was already thinking that I would not be concerned about losing it.

As the days passed slowly, I began again to write, and I wrote and sent out the newsletter in which I announced to the world that I had Cancer. I had started writing my newsletters telling about my personal life in 1998. Over the years, my newsletter readers' list had grown to include about sixty people. I usually wrote these newsletters at least one time every two weeks. Amazingly, even in the depths of my depression, I was able to write to my newsletter readers and tell them of my diagnosis. I wrote the following in that first announcement:

> I am sure that everything will be fine. Paul and I will make it through all of this together. I am more upset than he is. This just was *not* in my plans! I will prioritize my time now and choose more carefully where I spend my energies. I have so many wonderful friends that I know that I do not walk this road alone. My close friends here in Durango, my newsletter friends, my family, Paul's Phi Kappa friends, my Christ the

King family, and others will help me. I will get on with life simply because there is nothing else that I can do. I am a doer. I am active. I will go on.

I expressed hope and courage and gave some assurances to my supporters. Despite these encouraging words, inside I was shaking and barely holding myself together. I decided during this waiting time that I was going to wear my nice clothes anytime I wanted. It would be a shame to die and to leave all of my nice clothes in such good shape. No one would want my clothes, so I had better use them while I could. Before Cancer, I had only been wearing my nice clothes for Sundays or when I was going out or expecting company in.

During this time, I had to take the *big* step in the unplanned journey and my battle against Cancer. *I had to accept the fact that I had Cancer, and I had to somehow go on.*

Chapter 4

Ask Questions, Find Answers

Before my appointment that Thursday morning, July 17, to see the surgeon again, we stopped in at the Cancer Center in Durango. I didn't even know where this place was a couple of days ago. But my nurse friend, Marge, had encouraged us to look at it. We discovered that the center had a well-stocked Cancer library, and I checked out two books and picked up several free pamphlets. It looked like a nice place, but it was full of people who looked like they were dying. They all looked very sick. One lady we saw was in a wheelchair with an oxygen bottle. I surely did hope that I didn't get like that. These kinds of people are the really scary part of finding out that you have Cancer. This disease was going to make me face the fact that I was going to die. That fact was very hard for me to accept immediately.

In trying to learn about this disease, I had prepared a series of questions that I wanted to ask my doctor. I had them written on paper so that I could carry them in when I saw my doctor. I also carried a pencil with me so that I could jot down the answers. I will share them in this book because maybe they are questions that another breast Cancer patient may have. They were as follows:

Is my Cancer in stage 1, stage 2, or even a later stage?

> *The doctor told me that he would use blood tests, bone scans, CT scans, and x-rays to help him quantify my tumor. He could not stage it at this time. He knew, however, that it was going to be a stage 2 tumor or higher. I had learned from my studying that stages are a way of measuring the severity of a Cancer. Cancers are staged from a stage 1 to a stage 5. A stage 5 Cancer is very advanced, and one might die from this Cancer.*

BREAST CANCER: THE UNPLANNED JOURNEY - LESSONS LEARNED

The doctor explained that a stage 1 Cancer is a tumor that is three-fourths of an inch or less in size and that there are no lymph nodes involved, meaning that the Cancer has not spread beyond the breast.

A stage 2 Cancer is a tumor that is larger than three-fourths of an inch and has spread to some lymph nodes. The survival rate at this time in stage 2 Cancer is 80 percent in the 5-10 year range.

A stage 3 Cancer involves a tumor that is more than two inches in size.

He speculated that if the next surgery showed that the tumor was not bigger and that no lymph nodes were involved, my Cancer would be declared T2, N0, and MX. T2 means that its size is a stage 2, N0 means that there are no lymph nodes that show Cancer, and MX means that they didn't check the metastasis. Metastasis means that the Cancer has spread to any other parts of the body.

Do I have in situ carcinoma in both breasts?

The doctor told me that I probably did have it in the other side. However, he would not know for sure until he sent tissue from my left breast into the lab for analysis.

I had read on one of the research sites that if the Cancer tumor is located beneath the nipple, a mastectomy is preferable. I asked my surgeon if he recommends a mastectomy since my lump was right under the nipple.

The surgeon told me that he didn't know anything about this rule. He told me that he recommends another lumpectomy. He thought that he would get all of the Cancer in his second surgery.

I asked how many lymph nodes would be removed in the sentinel node biopsy that was planned.

The doctor told me that he would take out as many lymph nodes as he felt was necessary. He explained that if the Cancer had spread to more than three lymph nodes that it had probably spread in my body. He would recommend hormonal treatment and chemotherapy if I had more than three lymph nodes involved with Cancer.

I asked him about how we could find out if the Cancer had spread outside the lymph nodes.

He explained that when the Cancer spreads outside of the lymph nodes, it is called metastasis. He told us that there was a Cancer antigen test that is very similar to the one that is done for prostate Cancer. However, when they do this test for the breast, they don't know where the Cancer could have spread to. Therefore, it isn't effective. He said that blood tests were just not sensitive enough to be good with breast Cancer. He said that the way that he practiced with his patients was to do careful follow-ups. If anyone had soreness or pain somewhere that was not explainable, then he would suspect Cancer and check it out.

Will I get Lymphodema after the lymph node removals? (*Lymphodema* is a condition in which the cells cannot get rid of fluids. It occurs when lymph nodes in an area have been removed. With breast Cancer, lymphodema occurs usually in the arm.)

Dr. Dover didn't think that lymphodema was a real problem with his patients. He indicated that my worries were totally unfounded. His patients usually did not suffer with lymphodema. Paul and I both got good feelings from him on this issue.

I asked if the lymph node removal would complicate my recovery.

He indicated that I would have a drain and some extra sutures after the surgery. The drain could probably be removed ten days after the surgery. He recommended that I plan a lighter schedule that allowed for naps in my recovery from this surgery.

I asked the doctor about what the radiation treatment would be like if I had to have it.

He told me that the usual radiation treatments are given every weekday for six weeks.

I asked him what the other therapy considerations would be.

He explained that the following things would determine my treatment regimen:

The size of the primary tumor.
Has the Cancer spread to my lymph nodes?
The hormone receptor status of the Cancer cells.
My age.
Are there other Cancer cells in my breasts?

I had read about nuclear grading, vascular invasion, and HER-2/neu tests, so I asked him about each one of them in my case.

> *He explained that nuclear grading is not applicable for lobular carcinoma, the kind of Cancer that I had. He said that vascular invasion was absent in his first lumpectomy. He explained that he had ordered an HER-2/neu test and that we would get results from the labwork in ten days.*

I asked him why the mammogram never showed my lump.

> *He said that he just didn't know.*

After patiently answering all of our questions, the surgeon told us that he recommended a second lumpectomy with breast conservation, followed by radiation. His office scheduled my follow-up lumpectomy five days later on Monday, July 21. To get ready for this surgery, Dr. Dover scheduled a chest x-ray, a sonogram on the left breast, an EKG, and extensive blood tests. We went to the hospital that afternoon and did our precheck-in and all of the prescribed tests.

Because we had been busy and distracted all day, I classified this day as an "up" day. I hadn't had time to worry about myself. Learning is always an exciting experience for me. I had a lot to learn about the conditions that put me on this unplanned journey. *Facts served to better arm me for the fears and the trials ahead.*

Chapter 5

USE OTHERS' SUPPORT, BUT WATCH OUT FOR THE NEGATIVE

Waiting for Another Surgery

We went home, and I sat quietly to wait. I quit all of my volunteer jobs. I just didn't want to go out or to be bothered with peripheral things. I walked through life without feeling. Food had no flavor, and time seemed to march on independently, just dragging me along behind. I began to have my first "learning" experiences with how to deal with Cancer on a daily basis. For example, how do you answer the question, "How are you?"

I guess the first time I went out after getting the Cancer news was on Saturday, July 19, to our Women Helping Others (WHO) Charity Garden Tour. Since I am the WHO chairperson in Durango, I figured that I should probably attend this event. A group of friends and I met to go together to see the gardens. We had some amazingly beautiful gardens in this dry desert town to view that day. At one of the houses, one of my friends that I hadn't seen in a while came up to me, greeted me, and then innocently asked, "How are you?" My answer up until that day had always been, "I'm just fine, thank you. How are you?" Well, I was anything *but* fine. However, what do you say when you are asked this mundane everyday question?

I paused a moment before replying, and my friend answered the question for me by saying, "I bet you are really hot." That was a good answer. He hadn't really wanted to know how I was. He had been just making conversation. He wanted a casual answer, not the real one. I had just never before thought about this simple question and its implications in my life now. Answering this simple question was a real lesson in learning how to deal with life with Cancer.

I decided that it was best if I didn't truthfully answer all questions. I needed to evaluate my questioners and give them the answer that they expected. It wasn't good to overwhelm them, scare them off, or burden them with the real way that I felt that day or even later. *Casual friends don't really want to know how you are when you are dealing with a devastating diagnosis of Cancer.*

Support from All

Soon the word went out that I had breast Cancer. People that I had never even met before started emailing and calling me. They were Cancer survivors. They wanted to tell me their stories, and I wanted to listen. They were always supportive and encouraging. They gave me their phone numbers and promised to help any way that they could. I took notes and hoped, when hearing each one of their stories that my story would end happily also. I collected quite a few Cancer stories that I jotted down in my notebook. As I was writing this book, it was interesting to note and remember who called and how they are doing today.

People started sending me flowers, bringing food to our house, and coming by to visit. All of this was really nice. We didn't need the food. Paul cooks as well as I do, but it was nice to occasionally have someone else's food. I had always taken food to other people. I had always helped others in a "hard time." This was a real awakening to me to realize that I must be in a really "hard time" because I was now the recipient of these gifts and kindnesses. I enjoyed all of the visits, the cards, the e-mails, and the calls. Everyone wanted to help, but I didn't know how they could. I alone had to deal with this monster that had somehow gotten into my body.

A Very Sad, Bad Cancer Tale

Just a day or two after I had found out that I had Cancer, one of my neighbors whom I will simply call Jane that I thought was a friend came over and spent the morning with me. She told me that her mother had undergone a double mastectomy and had started her battle with Cancer many years ago when my neighbor, Jane, was only fourteen. Jane was now in her fifties, so Jane's mother was diagnosed with Cancer a long time ago. Her mother was stoic and didn't share her pain and suffering with her children or her husband. Jane's mother's marriage fell apart after her mastectomy, and she died a lonely, bitter, blaming lady—a sad victim of breast Cancer.

Jane that day was my angel of gloom. She predicted in warning tones that I would nearly be disabled after this surgery and would not be able to climb the stairs in our house. She predicted that Paul and I would probably be forced to move into a downstairs bedroom because of the lymph-node surgery that I was going to have. She told us that I would need help in putting on my clothes because I wouldn't be able to move my arms very much. In a loving tone, she told me that she had experienced this kind of surgery with her mother and just wanted to prepare me for what lay ahead.

Jane proceeded on with her black story and told me that Paul and I would have to communicate with each other in order to keep our marriage together. She further explained that after her mother's mastectomy, her mother had not wanted to be touched, and her father had not understood. Jane and her mother had been very close, and when her mother died, Jane somehow felt responsible. She had always felt like it was her responsibility to take care of her mother and that she had failed. Jane read that day a deathbed letter from her mother that she had found after her mother's death. The letter was written to all of the children (a sister, my neighbor, and a younger brother). It was a sad and beautiful letter. Jane's mother ended up dying from an impacted colon. It sounded like she had a horrible death. The conversation and the prediction of dark times ahead sent me tumbling into despair.

My friend had experienced a really difficult time and had lots of issues concerning her mother's death that she had never worked out. This "enlightenment of a terrible Cancer experience" was a horrible thing for "my friend" to give to me. Somehow Jane thought that she was helping me. Instead she was pushing me further down into that awful hole that I had fallen into when the doctor told me that I had Cancer. I should have been strong enough to stop "my friend" when she started this awful tale, but I didn't even try. She used my new Cancer as an opportunity for her to unburden her soul about the guilt and the problems that she had with her mother's death. I suppose that telling her story helped her, but it surely didn't help me.

Watch out for "friends" who remind you of the bad things that often come from Cancer. Cancer treatments have improved dramatically in the years since Jane's mother contracted the disease. Her experiences weren't really applicable to me at this time. However, when Jane told me the story, the death due to Cancer felt very real and was horrifying to me. At this stage in the unplanned journey, I needed to think and hear about how people had beaten Cancer—how they had survived. I was desperately trying to find things that I could grab on to so that I wouldn't fall farther down into depression. I had already seen my mother-in-law, Lillian Hyde, die a sad and painful death in 1983 that started from breast Cancer. Right now, a dear lady (Sandy) in our church was dying from Cancer that had spread from her breast to her lungs and her bones. I really did not want to get into either of those two situations. I just hoped and prayed that I would not have to endure a death from Cancer.

Just Getting By

In one of my newsletters at this time, I wrote the following:

> I have been so involved with this dreaded disease that I can't make myself sit down and write. The battle against Cancer is all-consuming. I don't have any energy or emotion left for anything else. Poor Paul lives here and helps and cares for me but gets little or nothing from me. I just seem to exist.

I found myself living in a horrible limbo land while I waited for this second lumpectomy. I just "got through each day" and that was absolutely all. I had no energy for anything but Cancer and the decisions, the surgeries, and the healings that I was involved in. I cried and cried and cried. In fact, I wore myself out crying. On Saturday, July 19, I decided that it was time for me to stop feeling sorry for myself; to accept that I had this awful, dreaded disease; and to get on with my life, which at this point would be battling Cancer. On Sunday, before the second lumpectomy, I wrote in my journal the following:

> *This was another bad day. This crying just absolutely wears me out. I have to somehow figure out how not to do this. I cannot continue to cry and cry and cry. I just wish that I knew that this Cancer was not a horrible death sentence. Facing one's death is hard. I always thought that I would live to be 104. I guess that I overestimated things. I sincerely hope that I do not die a long, drawn-out, painful, debilitating Cancer death. I haven't found anyone yet who has had a tumor that is as large as mine. That is scary. Everyone else's Cancer growths were small compared to mine.*
>
> *Surgery is tomorrow. Soon, maybe we will know what we are dealing with. I surely would feel better if I knew what was ahead.*
>
> *Sleeping tonight is hard. Paul and I are both awake. I woke up at 12:30 a.m, and it is now after 2:00 a.m. We are both nervous about tomorrow. I am not really nervous about the surgery. I think that Dr. Dover is an excellent surgeon. I am very nervous about the outcome and the diagnosis.*

Chapter 6

Life and Plans Go On—Go with the Flow

Another Surgery

Monday morning, July 21, we went to the hospital at six. This time, the surgery was a little more formal. I had two good friends from my Stephens Ministry group, Paul and Jigger Staby, who came to the hospital to be with Paul and me. I lay in the surgery ready room, in my hospital gown, on my gurney. It was comforting to hear that Paul Staby had endured a terrible liver Cancer from which he thought that he might die. However, he recovered and was then an eight-year survivor. I had known him for several years and hadn't known that he also had battled Cancer.

However, before I received the anesthetic that would knock me out for the surgery, the doctor came in and gave me a shot in my right breast near the lumpectomy. He injected a radioactive fluid. This shot hurt, but the hurt only lasted a very short time. The doctor had to give this shot to me two hours before the surgery so that it would have time to run into my body and lymph nodes. Later, the doctor gave me a shot of blue dye in the same area. I was already asleep when this shot occurred. These two substances would allow the surgeon to locate the lymph nodes that might be infected with Cancer. These two things were critical parts of my sentinel node biopsy.

The anesthesiologist came in and talked to me right after I had received the radioactive fluid shot. He asked if I was susceptible to motion sickness, and I told him that I was. He thought that was what probably had caused my vomiting when I was coming out from the sleeping medications during my last surgery (a rectal repair done in October 2001). He put a patch behind my ear to combat this motion sickness. He also gave me a Pepcid so that I wouldn't have any acid reflux. He promised that he would stay right with me throughout the operation.

As he started to put me under, Jigger asked that we pray, and we all prayed. That prayer was the last thing that I remembered before I went to sleep at 8:00 a.m. I didn't wake up until 2:00 p.m. Paul said that I had come out of the surgery at 1:00 p.m. The surgery lasted a lot longer than the one and a half hours of predicted time.

BREAST CANCER: THE UNPLANNED JOURNEY - LESSONS LEARNED

Dr. Dover got into the old cut on my breast and had cut out one more centimeter of flesh around the edge of where the tumor had been. He cut under my arm to look at the lymph nodes. He found one that was really obviously full of Cancer, and he cut this one out and did a frozen biopsy. The biopsy came back positive from the pathology lab. He then took out the four sentinel nodes and a three-inch diameter fat bed that contained the lymph nodes behind this infected lymph node. I suspected that he had taken out all of the auxiliary lymph nodes from my right arm. I hoped that I wouldn't have trouble with fluid collection in my arm (lymphodema).

This time they did not bandage me up tightly like they had done on the first surgery because of my allergic reaction to the tape. I wore a tight medical bra that was soft and much more comfortable than the tight taping had been. I felt a little more soreness than I had felt after the first lumpectomy, but I was all right. I went home that afternoon, had a good supper, and lay down to watch TV. However, I went to sleep very deeply before I had watched even one show, and therefore, I didn't take my pain medicine at 10:00 p.m. like I should have. At 2:00 a.m., I awoke in very bad pain. I woke Paul to help me, and I took my pain pills. *One should not get behind the pain curve.* It took a while for the pain medication to take effect. Paul fussed at me for not being more faithful in following the pain-pill regimen.

After this surgery, I had a drain tube and a collection bulb hanging from the lymph-node wound. The fluid that collected in this bulb had to be changed, and the quantities had to be measured and written down every few hours. Paul had to take care of this procedure at first.

Since I was not feeling up to par, Paul took all of my calls and sent out e-mails updating everyone about the surgery that I had just had. Paul was a good caregiver, and I was very lucky to have had him with me. I quickly started to get over the worst part of this second lumpectomy, and I felt that we were moving on down the road in getting rid of my Cancer. I had to recover, and we anxiously awaited the results of the pathology report. Dr. Dover came with excellent credentials, and we felt sure that he had removed all the Cancer from my breast this second time. Unfortunately, the Cancer had spread out of my breast into my lymph nodes. I would have to undergo chemotherapy and other corrective treatments.

Hosting My High School Class Reunion

In 2002 long before I knew that I was going to be battling Cancer, I agreed to host our next high school class reunion. The McCamey High School Class of 1961 Reunion had been scheduled for July 25, 26, and 27, in Durango. A week before this event, I announced to my classmates that I had Cancer. I explained about my lumpectomies, but I assured everyone that I would be all right. I secretly knew that Paul could take over hosting this affair if I needed him to. I explained that the reunion would proceed as scheduled. I welcomed them all. Sixteen of my classmates and their spouses were planning to attend. I had been making plans and working on preparations for it all year. I wanted nothing to ruin this event for my very good friends. I wanted life to go on as normal as possible.

On Friday, July 25, the old crowd started arriving. I had set up my orange and black table using our school colors and had put out all of my old annuals and scrapbooks on the table for viewing. We sat in our nice front yard in the shade, visited, and reminisced about times in McCamey, Texas, in the late 1950s and the early 1960s.

Paul cooked hamburgers at our house that evening. We had lots of fun activities scheduled, including the train ride up to Silverton and back, but I just didn't have the energy to participate in most of them. I really treasured seeing and visiting with my old friends, however. As a hostess, I did just what was required, nothing more. Paul filled in for me on the outings, and my wonderful friends cooked and helped around the house. It was not my best time. I gladly took the help that was freely given from all.

Monday, July 28, from My Diary

It has been seven days now after my second lumpectomy. My surgeon did not receive the pathology reports from the lab today. My drain is still draining too much fluid for it to be removed. I think that we are beginning to figure out how to handle my pain, however. I do not take enough pain medicine, and when I get to hurting, I get very depressed. When I don't hurt too badly, I am much more upbeat and able to handle things. Paul has decided that he is going to take over my pain management and plans to give me pain medication for a while. Two Advils keep me fairly comfortable. However, it seems right now that I must take them regularly. My pain level from the last surgery is still quite high.

My McCamey High School class reunion went quite well, considering that I was the host and had absolutely no energy. One of my classmates, Sherry Babcock Phillips, came early on Thursday afternoon so that she could help me. Everyone else helped also. One of my friends, Sandra Bradshaw Kurtin, and her mother, Marzelle Bradshaw, stayed with me. They did work around the house and changed their sheets and cleaned their rooms perfectly when leaving. I really enjoyed seeing and visiting with everyone. However, I did not do anything with the group except to sit around my own house. Paul took them on the train to Silverton on Saturday. I stayed home and slept. I went with the group that evening to the Bar-D-Chuck Wagon. However, I couldn't sit through the whole program. I had to get up and leave. Sunday, Paul took the group to Mesa Verde, and again I stayed home. Everyone left about midnight on Sunday evening. Of course, I was already in bed asleep. But the reunion is done! I did not want to cancel it and ruin people's vacations. I will rest this week until we get the pathology reports. I have received flowers, cards, food, and numerous calls from lots of people. I am well supported, loved, and prayed for. I have talked to a lot of Cancer survivors. Some of the women had big tumors that were seemingly cured for now. I may go to the Cancer support group here tomorrow night. I certainly do not want to do this awful Cancer battle alone. I need help.

I hope that I am done with the surgeries. My breast is the ugliest thing that I have ever seen—black, blue, yellow, red. The cut under my right arm is ragged, sore, and swollen.

Life went on, and somehow I managed to go on with it. I was glad that I had not canceled the reunion. I was glad that the second lumpectomy was over. I had spent several days enjoying my very good friends. Now my energies could be spent making my walk on the unplanned journey, fighting Cancer.

Chapter 7

FOLLOW THE DOCTOR'S DIRECTIONS, ESPECIALLY IN PAIN MANAGEMENT

Pain Management

I continued learning how to handle life with Breast Cancer. The immediate lesson that I was working on was pain management. I began to think that the word *Cancer* meant the same thing as *pain*. I had lived my whole life virtually pain free until then. I think that I had been awfully lucky. My philosophy on pain had been to "never admit that you have it," and it will probably go away before too long.

Before Cancer, I had lived that philosophy quite successfully. Even through two surgeries in 2000 and 2001, this philosophy had worked pretty well. The surgery in 2000 (a bladder tack and a hysterectomy) was pretty rough, but I healed quickly so I was able to "tough it out" through the first days of home recovery. The rectal repair that I had in 2001 was very easy, and I was able to handle the pain from it handily. However, Cancer surgeries seemed to be more than I could handle. I wrote in my diary about my pain and said:

> I think that I am accepting that I am in a different situation now than I have ever been in before. I don't like it, but it isn't fun to hurt all the time either.

When Paul would ask me how I felt each morning, my standard answer was fine. I always lied and pretended that everything was "hunky-dory". However, one morning, Wednesday, July 30, the first day that I had felt good at all, I answered his usual morning question truthfully. I told him that it felt like someone had taken a big five-foot car towing chain and had given me a big whack across my right breast and arm. All of a sudden, his eyes got as big as saucers and he looked at me like, "What's wrong with you this morning?" *Being honest about my pain was not always good, but I needed to learn to be more open with my partner.* I had to work on it to find the right words.

Anyway, after Paul got over his shock, we talked truthfully about how I felt. I had not been sleeping well at night because my body hurt in the bed. No matter how I turned, something hurt. I felt sharp burning pains down in my boob, in my chest under my arm, and even in the high muscles of my right arm and shoulder. My right breast was swollen and hard and heavy. It was black, blue, yellow, and red. My pain level did not seem to be decreasing each day. After other surgeries, when the pain was diminishing each day, I was able to endure it, knowing that I was getting better. With this second lumpectomy, I did not seem to be improving daily, so I figured that I had better learn to deal with the pain.

After much discussion and some arguing, Paul and I agreed that I really needed pain medicine on a continual and regular basis. So I began to take a daily regimen of Advil. This new pain management routine greatly helped my spirits and my coping abilities. I began sleeping longer at night, without waking up from pain. I still could not sleep through the night, however. I was like a baby. I had to have my regular night feeding of painkillers, but I was taking them, and as a result, I was resting much better than I had been doing before.

After I had read the doctor's surgical notes, I could understand a little better why I was still hurting. He did a lot of deep cutting into my breast tissues and into the muscles under my arm. When one is fighting Cancer, normal healing does not always occur. I had to learn about my own pain management. *You can't "tough it out" with Cancer*. It was a hard lesson for me, but hopefully I had learned this lesson now and would be better equipped to handle my next surgeries on the unplanned journey.

I had learned that I *must* take pain medicines for as long as they are needed (not for just a day or two like I think the dosage should be). I wasn't sure how I would know that it was okay to stop the medication, but my nurse friend, Marge, told me that I would know. She felt guilty about my problem and told me that if insurance companies hadn't taken over the world of medicine with their standardized allowances and definitions of what was needed, I would have stayed in the hospital for about five days following this surgery. In the hospital, the nurses would have helped me manage my pain, and things would have gone better. She is a *dear* friend, and I missed her smiling face and her sage advice when I was away from her in Texas.

Surgery Recovery

I was taking my pain medicine pretty regularly every six hours at this time. I was also taking two Advils with each meal. Even with visitors in our house, I slept most of the afternoon. I made the following inscription in my diary on Tuesday afternoon:

> I didn't cry much today. I hope that the waterworks are over. I am pretty sore. I am wearing my arm in a sling. Something really stings under my arm if I do much with it. My other cuts on my breast hurt also if I do not take the pain medicine. Everyone is really kind and sweet to me. I think that I have accepted that I have a bad Cancer

now. I do think that it is not too bad to "fix," however. It really has ruined our summer plans. Today was a pretty good day. I stayed home all day, but people came to visit and I talked a lot on the phone.

More Bad News

Tuesday evening, the doctor called with the pathology report from my surgery. One of the four sentinel nodes that he had removed had been Cancerous. One of the eleven other lymph nodes had a few Cancer cells in it. The pathology report indicated that he still had not gotten clear margins. The results from the pathology slides were not available for him to check at the time of the surgery. He made an appointment for me to come in and see him the next day, Wednesday, July 30.

I woke up and felt good on Wednesday, July 30, 2003, for the first day since my surgery nine days before. My head felt clear. My pain level was down. I felt like there might be a little hope in the world. I worked around the house. We saw my surgeon. We had been thinking about transferring to MD Anderson Cancer Center in Houston. Knowing that my surgeon had completed two lumpectomies and had not gotten all of the Cancer out of my breast, we decided that we must make the change and the move.

I wrote that evening, expressing some of my fears and frustrations as follows:

> I guess that I will learn the rules of this battle as I go along. I surely do hate to be on this road. I know well that I do not have the strength to do this battle alone. I need lots of help, and fortunately, I have it. I know that God has a plan for this disease and for me. I don't think that God gave me this trouble. I do not want to walk this road or to be in this battle against Cancer, but I do not have a choice. On the good days, I feel that everything will be all right. I can talk about it now without crying all of the time. I think that I have finally hit the bottom of the hole. Now maybe I can start the long climb back out. This is one of the hardest things that I have ever had to do. I have many, many good friends and family members who are right there with me. I will make it, but, gee whiz, it is hard!

Chapter 8

CAREFULLY KEEP YOUR RECORDS—MEDICAL AND PERSONAL

Medical Records

Very soon after I found out that I had Cancer, I began to keep a medical notebook with all of the doctors' reports and lab tests in it. This source of information that I carried with me became very helpful. By being able to read the reports myself, I was able to increase my understanding and knowledge beyond just what the doctors told me. I didn't know it at the time but I now believe that everyone should always have his medical records in his hands. The doctors in different places weren't good at getting all of the records that they needed. It seemed that during this journey, I had to go to many different doctors and hospitals. It is not difficult to obtain one's records. At the doctors' offices, you have to simply fill out and sign the correct forms. Usually the office personnel will then just copy the records for you. However, in some offices you have to wait for the records to be copied and then mailed to you. At the hospitals, you have to go to the records department, fill out the correct forms, and then wait to pick up the records.

When I first tried to get my medical records at MD Anderson after my first surgery there, I had to hunt for the medical records department. I was amazed to find that in this huge hospital complex that services thousands of people each day, the medicals records room was about the size of a very small closet. There was only one lady inside. I filled out a form, and within ten minutes I was holding the twenty-five pages of my records (from this first surgery and first examination and tests). I couldn't believe obtaining my records was simple and easy. This was another example of how MD Anderson's methods were very efficient and complete.

My medical notebook grew as time went by, and I went further on the unplanned journey. I still keep the book and find it to be very handy. It is quite thick now and needs to be divided into two big notebooks. The secret to using this collection of medical records is to be very organized and to keep a detailed index. When I come into a doctor's office with this big book, everyone is overwhelmed. I have to explain to them that I do not expect them to ever look at this notebook. I assure them that I will find and locate any of my medical information that is needed. When they ask for something and I easily locate it in this thick filing system, they are happy and impressed. I keep things that are alike together under one tab. For example, blood tests and urine tests are under one tab sorted by dates. Each doctor that I see has his own tab and each hospital stay has a separate tab. My index now covers several pages because there are many tabs. My notebooks are now very heavy to transport, but they are very useful and valuable.

I have found that consecutive test records, such as EKGs, blood tests, and pathology reports, just do not make their way from medical facility to medical facility. My medical notebook has saved me hours of time and gives the doctors and nurses accurate and complete information. You must be religious about going back to each doctor and each hospital and signing the needed papers in order to get copies of all of your records. This record collection so far has not cost me any money but has saved me several additional medical tests and, of course, money because medical tests that I already had completed did not have to be redone. Someday all of our records will be electronic and will be available to all medical personnel. But until that day comes, it is to your advantage to have paper copies or disks of your records in your hand.

Your Personal Support Records

At this time, I also began keeping all of the beautiful and comforting cards that I received. Quickly the quantity became too large to handle easily so I put all of them into a big manila envelope that I planned to carry with me. I began to keep all of my supportive e-mails in a Word folder that I hoped to print out and to put into a notebook later. Further down the road, when Paul and I were in Houston, away from our loving and supporting friends, I thought that I might need to read these earlier missives of hope and help again. I felt that reading these cards would help me feel supported when I got blue and down.

I didn't know that I was going to keep on receiving a loving supply of these cards. As time went on, I had too many lovely cards to carry in my manila envelope. I soon had to devise another system. I ended up not carrying my cards with me when I went to the hospital in Houston as I had earlier planned. I filed them in a picture storage box alphabetically. I kept this box by my chair in the living room in our small apartment so that I could read and file my cards each day. I now have a large card file of beautiful "get well' cards that I take out and look at every once in a while. Some friends sent me many cards. I will always treasure this physical proof of my support during my Cancer battle. It was always there when I needed it when I had a particularly difficult day. It was full of reminders of love and prayers sent by my army of supporters. It was proof that I wasn't alone in this journey.

Chapter 9

Find Good Models—Cancer Survivors

It was good for me when I was deep into this unplanned journey to look around for some heroes that I could learn from and mirror. Anyone who is setting off on a Cancer adventure should read and study how other people have successfully made the trip. I kind of did this at the very first of my adventure when so many Cancer survivors called me to tell me their stories. However, now that I was deeper into the battle, I needed more information and more inspiration. I read several books, one of which was written by a lady doctor, Amy Givler, who had Cancer of the lymph nodes (a kind of lymphoma). It was entitled *Hope in the Face of Cancer, A Survival Guide for the Journey You Did Not Choose*. It was fairly good and offered some interesting pointers for me. However, it did not satisfy my hunger for inspiring models.

My sweet new daughter (my daughter-in-law, Liz Dittmer, wife of our number one son,) gave me Lance Armstrong's book *It's Not about the Bike, It's about Getting Back My Life*. I couldn't put this inspiring book down. I completed it in only a few days. My soul was hungry for a winning story of stamina and strength against very bad odds with Cancer. Lance Armstrong, in his first book, gave me that story. Lance's Cancer story, even though it was not breast Cancer, gave me real hope of beating the monster Cancer and of returning to a normal life.

Armstrong effectively described the overwhelming feelings that accompanied his diagnosis of Cancer and how the diagnosis overturned everything in his life. He described how, as the doctors studied more completely the case and his condition, things just got worse and worse. To top everything off, he didn't have medical insurance either. He was too sick to work or to race. His Cancer was very aggressive and had nearly taken over his body. How would he handle things? I was so engrossed in Lance's story that I literally devoured the book. I wanted to see how Armstrong "beat" his Cancer and returned to a full life. I could hardly put it down to eat or to sleep. I hoped that I could surely do what Lance had done since my prognosis was much more positive than his had been. I knew, however, that I was not as tough or as strong as he was. His book was most enjoyable. It was a stimulating book that encouraged me. I had a real need at this time in my life to hear happy Cancer-survivor stories.

BREAST CANCER: THE UNPLANNED JOURNEY - LESSONS LEARNED

I needed to read inspiring books, and I looked everywhere for examples of people who had beaten their Cancers. I hoped that I could be as strong in my battle against Cancer as Lance and some of my other models had been. I hope that my book will add to your knowledge and encourage you. My Cancer was difficult, but I made it through it, and my life is now good.

Chapter 10

STORE MEMORIES OF STRENGTH AND HAPPINESS

MD Anderson Appointment

When Dr. Dover did not remove all of the Cancerous cells during my second lumpectomy, my doctor daughter advised me that it was time to move my treatment to the MD Anderson Cancer Hospital in Houston, Texas. My family was very happy with this decision to transfer my medical care back to Texas because I would be a little closer to them. I had gotten on the Internet and had found the MD Anderson site, http://www.mdanderson.org. It was easy to navigate through, and I quickly found the application for admittance that I filled out, saying that I had Cancer and wanted treatment at MD Anderson. I finished this form on my computer and sent it back to MD Anderson as an e-mail. It was all very quick and easy. Within twenty-four hours of my completing this task just as the directions had indicated, a person called me from Houston. He was to be my personal representative at MD Anderson. He asked me lots of questions and told me what I needed to do. He was able to make appointments for me and everything. I was amazed that it was so easy to get into this renowned Cancer center.

At this time, everything seemed to be set at MD Anderson. The doctor in Durango had faxed my medical records to Houston. I had my mammogram films and my sonogram stuff in my hands to take with me. I had worked with the lab in Durango, and they would be overnighting my pathology slides as well as specimen blocks from my lump to the labs at MD Anderson. My first appointment with the MD Anderson surgeon was scheduled for August 14. I was eager to hear what MD Anderson would say about my Cancer.

BREAST CANCER: THE UNPLANNED JOURNEY - LESSONS LEARNED

Last-Minute Tasks

Hopes and Help

After making the decision to leave Durango and go to Houston, we had to get ready to move. It had been nine days since I had undergone a second lumpectomy. My physical condition was improving. I could feel that I was still recovering. I took a nap around lunchtime each day. I didn't lift things with my right arm. I hoped that by the time that we got to Houston to see the doctor again, my surgeries would be close to being healed. I hoped that the pain would have lessened also. I continued with my pain management (taking Advil regularly) for a while longer.

I had to gather and to store all of the memories of my friends and supporters in Durango. Seeing them and saying good-bye took just about all of the energy that I had at that time, but I set about to complete these enjoyable tasks.

One of my friends, Ginna Harbison, came to visit me and pointed out that our tears were just pressure-relief valves like the ones that are found on pressure cookers. The tears we shed right now are just releasing the pressure from the fears and the things that we had cooking inside of us. I guess that she was right. At least now I wasn't crying all of the time. I am sorry to say that about a year later, Ginna was diagnosed with two Cancerous growths in one breast and even another growth in her other breast. She too had to battle Cancer. We just didn't know what lay ahead for either of us at the time of that last meeting in 2003.

I had gotten cards and e-mails, some of which came from people that I didn't even know. I had gotten prayer notifications from churches that I had never been to. It certainly was gratifying and encouraging knowing that I had so many people pulling for me in this battle. I was dragged and pushed down the first quarter mile of this road of battling Cancer, but I was now on the road of this unplanned journey, and I would walk it to the end. Everything would somehow be okay.

I was very thankful that Paul walked beside me. He was always there for me to lean on when I needed him. He was busy at this time, packing our things in preparation for our leaving Colorado. I didn't know how this trip back to Texas was going to go, but I was trying very hard to let him do the packing and the planning. I felt that we would somehow find our way. I felt thankful to everyone for helping us.

My Writing E-mail Lists

As we closed down our Colorado residence and said good-bye to our many friends, I discovered that I now had a dilemma to handle. I had started an email "Cancer Update List" of people who had expressed the desire to keep up with my well-being. The people on this list regularly received short notes about what was happening with my Cancer. I already had an old list of people who received my weekly newsletters that I had written since 1998. A lot of my friends ended up being on both of these lists. This hadn't been a problem at the beginning of this journey because at first, I just stopped writing my regular weekly newsletters. But now that I seemed better able to handle things and began to write my newsletters again, I didn't know who to send them to. When the dam broke on my newsletter writing blockage, the writings just seemed to come pouring from my computer. I decided that it was time to just ask all of my friends who were on the "Cancer Update List" if they wanted to be included in my "Newsletter List" also.

The two missives had different purposes. The Cancer Update that I ended up writing nearly daily was short (limited to absolutely one page) and just gave the facts about my medical condition. My newsletter, which I ended up writing nearly weekly, was usually long and told what I felt and what I was thinking about my condition and about my life. I gave people a choice as to which list that they wanted to be on. If they wanted both of the writings, I included them on both lists. I pointed out that if I got especially ill or depressed, I might not write the newsletters. However, Paul or I would always try to write the Cancer updates. I mentioned that friends who subscribed to my newsletter would receive the full picture of my life. They would get the interesting stories about my special kitty, Mr. Boots.

I ended up with two different lists. All of the newsletter subscribers opted to get the Cancer updates, but everyone on the Cancer Update List did not want to receive my newsletters. I just wanted to be able to write and to keep my friends and family happy and updated. It is because of all of this writing that I did as we traveled down this road of the unplanned journey that I am able four years later to sit down and to write this book. I would have forgotten too many of the details had I not had all of my earlier writings to refer to. Writing has always served as an emotional release for me. It serves to calm my fears and my soul.

Getting Ready to Leave

Doctor's Release

I saw my surgeon, Dr. Dover again on Wednesday, July 30. He checked things out and cleared me to travel to Texas. My breast only had a big gauze bandage over the lumpectomy spot. The wound was red, ugly, and swollen.

Shutting Down the Colorado Home

After we had made our decision to leave Colorado and to treat this Cancer at MD Anderson in Houston, Texas, our work seemed to be fairly straightforward. We began the work of shutting down the house. Plants had to be distributed to friends. We moved all of our outdoor furniture and miscellaneous equipment into the garage. Paul was in charge of this move, and I tried to do as he said. I rested a lot.

We made our plans to leave on Tuesday, August 5. Paul felt that I should fly to Texas to save the wear and the tear on my body from a two-day driving trip. Paul would drive back. He would carry my BeautiControl inventory, Mr. Boots (our special kitty), and his computer in our truck. I worried about him until he arrived safely at our home in Grapevine.

Saying Good-bye

Packing up and leaving Colorado was difficult. Saying good-bye to all of our Colorado friends was tough. I explained that I didn't think that we would return to Colorado until May or June of 2004. I would more than likely have further surgeries in Houston at MD Anderson. This would mean that I would be taking chemotherapy in the October through March time frame. It just didn't seem wise for us to come back to Colorado in the winter for me to undergo chemotherapy where the snow and cold temperatures sometimes made things difficult. It is usually absolutely lovely in Texas in the winter. I hoped to return to Colorado next spring when I was all healed and ready to live my life again.

We said good-bye to our many friends. I actually believed that some of them might come down to Texas that winter for a visit, but they didn't. I gave and received lots of hugs and promises that we would "stay in touch." I felt very close to these supportive friends. They are all wonderful folks that Paul and I loved, respected, and needed. Saying good-bye filled our time. I was working at storing up memories and pulling in strength from the people in Durango.

My Breast Condition

My diary on Sunday, August 3, included the following description of the condition of my right breast:

> The soreness in my right breast is finally lessening some. The extreme combination of discoloration is lightening. Only the front part of my breast is black now. The swelling has not reduced much, but things seem to be a little better overall. I still think that the breast is poisoned and needs to be removed.

> My right arm is still very sore. It probably hurts more than my breast. The cut is apparently healed under my arm, but the soreness inside my arm has not lessened much. This is the area that I need the pain medicine for. If I get out of pain medicine, this place still feels raw and newly cut. I wake up in the night to take more pain medication. It will be nice to make it through a night without waking one of these days. What a big step that would be!

Final Plans

I ended up flying out of Farmington, and Paul planned to drive me there (forty-five miles from our house) on Tuesday morning. Our wonderful, caring, and helpful neighbors, Delilah and John Orr, came over that last evening before we left to share dinner with us and to get the final instructions on the care of our house. They were fabulous and had agreed to water our plants, to watch our house, to turn the water off when cold weather arrived, and to complete the winterization process of our house after we left. What would we have done in Durango without our wonderful neighbors and friends?

Our friends, John and Therese Teiber, came over that evening also. We enjoyed a "last" visit with them filled with more good times. When everyone left, Paul and I went to bed with the alarm set for early the next morning. We were spending the last night in our beautiful Colorado home for quite a while. We didn't really know when we would get to come back.

The Departure Day Arrived, Leaving Colorado

Getting off and closing down a house is always a *big* job. This time, because of my weakness and pains, Paul did the job. It was difficult, and he really had a lot of work to do, but he got it done. We pulled out onto the highway at 9:15 a.m. (just fifteen minutes later than our plan). It was a perfect day, cool and sunny and bright. I tried to drink in the view of our La Plata Mountains as we drove toward Hesperus. I attempted to memorize the way that the Ponderosas (the variety of pine trees that were common in our yard and neighborhood) looked—all tall and green and majestic. I probably wouldn't see these giants again until next summer, and I thought that when I was tired and sick and weak, I would need to draw on these strong Colorado images for strength and courage.

I got on the plane in Farmington, and Paul drove off in our big red truck with Mr. Boots as his companion. The trip home for me was uneventful and fairly easy. I slept on the plane and enjoyed the sleep, except that I always got a crick in my neck from sleeping in a seat. I was tired when I got to the hot Dallas Fort Worth (DFW) airport, but I was fine.

Staying at Mary Lee's House

In Texas, my good friend and my daughter's mother-in-law, Mary Lee Hamisch, had insisted that she pick me up and take care of me. She met the plane and drove me to her house (which was clean and cool and operating). Our Texas house was "shut down," hot, and kind of dirty from having sat empty for the summer. Bugs always seemed to choose their dying places in the middle of our white tile floor when we were gone.

I spent my first evening in Texas in a very relaxed state eating a fabulous meal and visiting with Mary Lee. Mary Lee brought me up to date on the news from our kids. In Mary Lee's house, there was a wonderful large tub with water spray jets in it that she filled so that I could enjoy a long soaking tub bath before I went to bed. That night, I slept well and didn't wake up until 9:45 a.m. Mary Lee had gotten up before me but was very quiet. She fed me a delicious breakfast and drove me to my Texas house about 11:00 a.m. I couldn't have been pampered more than I was under Mary Lee's care. I really enjoyed my visit.

Joining the World of the Living Again

I took my last pain-relief medicine on Tuesday night at Mary Lee's house. I finally was able to go through the night without pain interrupting my sleep. That may have been one of the reasons that I slept so long and so well. I was joining the world of the "living" folks again. My pain level was down significantly. The drain hole that remained open since the doctor removed the plastic drain tube the previous Wednesday (July 30) had just about stopped draining gunk. I had been able to stop putting the big, thick "sop it up" bandages on the drain hole and could now put on just a regular Band-Aid. The burning, stabbing, raw pains that I had suffered from earlier had dulled to annoyances that I could bear. If I suddenly grabbed my right breast and a strange agonizing look covered my face, I told everyone not to worry. I was having one of those "healing" pains that occurred for short moments. Each pain would pass, and I was feeling so much better! I thought that I had passed through another trying time.

I was fourteen days out from my last surgery. I started to try to settle into our Texas house and to get everything going again. We were having record-breaking heat. That Tuesday, it was one hundred four degrees Fahrenheit, and that Wednesday, the day that I arrived, it was one hundred nine. Our air conditioner ran all of the time just to get the inside temperature down to eighty. Nudity should have been the accepted style of dressing in that kind of heat, although I couldn't let anyone see my ugly right breast.

It was also very dry in Texas. I thought that Paul might have lost his huge azalea plants that adorned our entrance courtyard. They had not been watered by rain, and they were struggling now. I immediately poured water on them after the plumber came and repaired the water turn-on valve. It had been hot and dry at our Texas house since we had left in June. Paul arrived in our big red truck that afternoon. He and Mr. Boots had made the trip without any trouble, and I was really glad to have them safe and with me again.

Chapter 11

LISTEN TO YOUR BODY

Life in Grapevine, Texas

Breaking a Solid Board with My hand

In 2001, I had decided that I would become a consultant for a skin care company named BeautiControl. This company has magnificent skin-care products, a full line of cosmetics, and other beauty and bath aids. I had agreed to sell these products because I liked them so well and wanted to be able to buy them at a discounted price. Their annual sales meeting was being held in Dallas, August 7, 8, and 9. I had planned to attend this meeting before I found out that I had Cancer. It was logical for me to still go because my MD Anderson appointment was not until August 14. I had the time.

On Thursday, I went to Dallas to attend this meeting with my neighbor, Marilyn Gunn, to hear the inspirational speaker that BeautiControl had scheduled for their first meeting. The man, Brian Biro, was a good speaker with a message saying that we could enrich our lives and reach fabulous goals if we just did a few simple things. To prove this to us, at the end of the meeting, all one thousand of us who were attending were asked to break a $12 \times 6 \times ¾$ inch solid board of pinewood.

The ushers at the meeting came out and gave each of us a piece of pine board. Brian told us to write on one side of the board the one thing that we had been struggling with. He wanted us to write the one thing that was holding us back and the things that it caused. The thing that I felt was holding me back was Cancer, so I wrote, "Cancer—pain, handicaps, death," on one side of my board. On the back side of the board, he instructed us to write what we would have if we conquered this bad thing. I wrote, "Love for all, health, strength, energy, new opportunities, a book, and possibilities." He also had us dedicate the breaking of this board to someone. I dedicated my breakthrough to James and Paul Damian two of my sons, who were having a serious conflict at the moment. I had secretly thought that maybe the reason that I had this Cancer was to draw my family back together again.

He then instructed us to leave our seats and to gather at the back of the big room, standing in a big circle. There were so many people that the circle was several people deep, but all of us could see. He started this final demonstration by choosing someone from the audience to break the first board. He chose a little lady who was standing beside her wheelchair. She wobbled out to the middle of the floor where Brian was. We all excitedly yelled and cheered words of encouragement. And amazingly with our support and Brian's instructions on the third try, this weak, handicapped woman pushed the sole of the palm of her bare hand through the board. I couldn't believe that she could do this, but I also couldn't believe that BeautiControl would be sponsoring a scam. They were an "honorable" company as far as I could tell. Were there "magical powers" in our minds? Were we able to harness these powers and to use them to do physical, real-world things? Could the mental support of others actually help us do physical things? I just didn't know. I certainly didn't think that I could break the solid board that I was holding in my hand.

After Brian's encouraging and inspiring talk and this dazzling board-breaking demonstration, we broke into smaller groups of about ten to twelve ladies and started breaking boards under the supervision of Brian's helpers. My next-door neighbor, Marilyn, who was not particularly strong, broke her board on the second try. She made it actually look easy. Brian was giving us a practical exercise in visualization to reality. Because of my surgery and the limited use that I had of my right arm, I felt that I had to try to break the board with my left arm. This was extremely difficult because my left arm is considerably weaker than my right arm. I was awkward using my left hand and had very limited strength on my left side. However, with Brian's instruction and help, I broke the board just like everyone else. It took me several tries, but somehow the board broke in half. I was flabbergasted. I surely didn't use my own visualization to reality to do this. I must have used everyone else's visualization.

I keep the broken board in a recipe-book holder stand on my bookshelves in my living room. It remains a constant reminder to me of the power of the mind over physical things. During the unplanned journey, I kept the broken board in my bright yellow ribbon-covered bag, where I kept my "get well" cards, a small Bible, my angel rock, and the special things that I wanted to keep with me when I underwent chemo. This broken board reminded me that I could do difficult things if I thought that I could and if I could overcome remembered practices. This was a positive experience of the power of the mind over matter. I was lucky to have gotten to participate in this seminar right at this time in my life when I would need all of my mental powers in this battle against Cancer.

The Consequences of My Not Listening to My Body

I was especially tired after the Thursday meeting. Marilyn drove me home from the Dallas meeting. I rested most of Friday. After a good nap in the afternoon, I decided that I would continue attending the BeautiControl (BC) meetings that evening. Attending was easy because my sweet neighbor, Marilyn, drove us to the Adams Mark Hotel that evening, about five, and we registered with thousands of other BeautiControl consultants. We checked in as roommates into a very luxurious room. We just had time to say hello to Marilyn's district director and to mine before we went down to the big opening meeting.

There were over three thousand BeautiControl consultants at this meeting. It was a big event for this small company that is a subsidiary of Tupperware. The stage in the front of the huge room was massive. The lights were bright, colorful, and dynamic. The music was loud and fast. There were several big screens at the sides of the stage, on which everyone could view with magnification the events and the people on the stage. This was a *real* company production. This was a "ra-ra" sales meeting. I had attended many of these when I worked for AT&T and NCR, but it was kind of nice to attend this one as a retired person. I didn't have work pressures on me now. My livelihood didn't depend directly on my sales anymore.

I enjoyed the talks, the people, and the excitement that levitated throughout the hall. A little after 9:00 p.m., however, I realized that I was very tired. I decided that I had enjoyed all of the sales meeting that I needed to. I explained to Marilyn that I was going up to our room, and I left the auditorium. I performed my "get to bed" routine leisurely, and thought to myself how nice it would be to spend a weekend with the girls in this nice hotel, not thinking about Cancer. I went to bed and managed to watch a TV show until 10:00 p.m., when I turned off the light. I was exhausted.

My breast had not gotten better and seemed to be getting worse since I had arrived in Texas. It was hard as a rock, was swollen so big that the outside skin was as tight as the covering of a snare drum. It was yellow and red colored where it had been black, and was hot to the touch. In "checking it out" that Friday afternoon before I left our house, I decided that it was probably going to bust, so I called my surgeon in Durango. Of course, he was tied up in emergency surgery. I knew that he would call me back when he could, so I gave Paul all of the instructions about my suffering breast and went on to my meeting. I was still excited from breaking that solid board and didn't want to miss any of the rest of the meetings.

My surgeon from Durango called about 9:00 p.m. (Texas time) and had forgotten that I was ino longer in Durango. Paul described my breast, and Dr. Dover suggested that I should see a doctor or go to the emergency room where we were "sooner rather than later." Paul took the directions but didn't try to call me or to pick me up. It was night, and he thought that things could wait until tomorrow.

It felt good to lie down in the hotel bed that night, but the bed wasn't comfortable. When your breast is the size of an overgrown softball or a cantaloupe, is hard as a rock, is very sore, and feels like it weighs twenty pounds by itself, it is hard to get into a comfortable position in the bed. However, I went immediately to sleep. I hadn't been asleep very long when it felt like something had hit and hurt my boob. It hurt awfully, and the pain shot through to my consciousness even though I was in a deep sleep. I was so exhausted, however, that I said to myself, "I do not want to wake up. This sleep is good. Stay asleep, Beverly." And I did.

My roommate, Marilyn Gunn, returned from the meeting a few minutes after twelve midnight. She tiptoed into our room, but I heard her. In this semi-awakening state, my hand brushed over my right side, and I felt wetness. I knew this wasn't normal, so I sat up and struggled to turn the light on. At the same time I called Marilyn's name. When I managed to find the light switch and to get the light on, she and I both saw that my right breast had been bleeding for a while. My bra and my nightshirt were soaked with blood. When I managed to sit upright, the blood just dripped from my shirt front. Marilyn let out a cry of anguish and immediately ran for the wash rags and the towels in our bathroom. I didn't actually make too much of a mess in the room beyond the bed, but what an experience! I bet the maids wondered if someone had been murdered in that bed. My right breast had simply burst while I was asleep and had continued to release its pressure by bleeding.

We put cold washrags on my bleeding breast, and I called Paul. Marilyn insisted that I stay in bed, and she set about to clean things up. Paul jumped into the car and drove the forty minutes to downtown Dallas to pick me up in the middle of the night. There wasn't any traffic on the roads to slow him down so he arrived quickly. I stuffed a wet towel over my bleeding breast and put on a clean surgical bra. Marilyn put some clothes over my head. I kept my right arm cradled against my chest inside of my clothes. I didn't even try to put my right arm through a sleeve. In the darkest and most alone time of the night, I went downstairs in downtown Dallas at the hotel to await Paul's arrival.

Marilyn was such a good and kind friend. She didn't get sick when I bled all over the bed, and she didn't scream or panic when she saw my ugly, engorged breast bleeding openly. She was pretty tough. She was a very dear friend to me that night. I am so thankful that she was with me. I might have really been scarred if I had been all alone in that hotel room. She was my lifesaver that night. Thank you, Marilyn.

We now knew what Dr. Dover's message, "Get her into medical care sooner rather than later," really meant.

Treating This New Condition

The Long, Dreary Drive Back to Grapevine

We decided to go to our neighborhood emergency room in Grapevine. We have Baylor Medical Hospital facilities in Grapevine and have always thought that they were quite good. We just drove right past the Dallas big hospitals. I didn't want to face a big-town emergency room on a Saturday morning at 1:00 a.m.

It was rather a long and cold drive back from Dallas that night, even though it was the middle of a hot summer. There were few cars on the road, and the lights of Dallas didn't really warm the night. I had known inside my head that my boob was going to blow up, but I had just not exactly known what to do about it. I should have gone to a doctor that Friday afternoon instead of going to my meetings. However, I do so hate to let a weak body rule my life. I want my mind and my spirit to rule my life and to just have my body follow along. I do so hate to be limited by my body. This Cancer thing had put my body in charge, and I hated that. I had just gotten off of the pain pills so that I thought my life was getting back a semblance of normalcy to it. I didn't want to have Cancer ruling everything I did again. I was very stubborn, but with this bout, I had lost. My stubbornness had done nothing but complicate and make my situation worse. Cancer had won this round.

I was leaving my planned meetings, I would miss the wedding that I so wanted to attend on Saturday, and I couldn't even imagine what else I had ruined. This was not a happy time for Paul or me. Paul loses patience with me when I act stubbornly and refuse to listen to my body. He cannot understand that I have always lived my life being controlled by my brain and my spirit. It was terribly hard for me to realize that in this battle with Cancer, I had to listen to my body. I had to let the needs of my body rule over my own mind. I had to arrange my activities around the cries and the desires of my body. My boob bursting was my fault, and it was difficult to accept what I had to learn from this incident. If I had listened to my body and had canceled my activities and had gone to see a surgeon in Grapevine that Friday afternoon, I do not believe that my breast would have burst. The surgeon would have gone in and would have drained the lumpectomy site and would have treated the infection. However, hindsight, as you know, is always so much clearer than foresight. Heed my advice if you are fighting a battle against Cancer—*listen to your body!*

A Saturday Morning Very Early in the ER

At 1:40 a.m., August 9, we pulled into the emergency room at Baylor Hospital in Grapevine. Within five minutes of our arrival, I was met by a triage nurse who evaluated my situation and determined that I was not dying or bleeding to death. After about an hour of waiting in an entrance room surrounded by crying, sleeping, injured people, we were taken back into the medical service area of the ER, to a curtained-off area (room) where I had a gurney to lie on. I was *not* a critical case, so Paul and I ended up waiting all night long.

Paul got awfully tired as he sat in the straight-back table chair that was the only sitting thing available in our area. I was at least lying down and could doze some, even though the gurney was hard. I was freezing also. I had a temperature, and the nurse would not let me have blankets. She didn't want to raise my temperature. I lay miserably on the hard gurney, shaking and feeling sorry for myself. Paul wouldn't leave my side, except for one time when he left for about twenty minutes to go home to put out a dirt box for Mr. Boots. I tried to get him to go out and to lie down in the car for a while, but he was afraid that he might miss seeing the doctor when he came, and so he sat miserably all night long.

My nurse looked at my breast and scared us. She said that it looked like that I had a bad infection. She thought for sure that the doctor would put me in the hospital to stay for a while. I anxiously explained that I had an appointment with a surgeon at MD Anderson in Houston on Thursday that I absolutely had to keep. She wasn't encouraging and didn't think that I would be out of Baylor in time to keep that appointment. The nurse put an IV in my arm but didn't hook it to anything. She drew blood for tests. She monitored my blood pressure and temperature all night while we waited for the doctor. It was a long, miserable, lonely night.

We waited until nearly morning before we finally saw the doctor. When the doctor got around to seeing me, he affirmed the nurse's diagnosis and said that I definitely had an infection of some kind. However, the drainage at this time appeared to be blood not pus. My highest temperature while I was in the ER was 99.6 degrees Fahrenheit, and my bloodwork showed normal white blood cell counts. The doctor prescribed a drip of a very strong penicillin, Augmentin. He gave me a prescription for the same medicine to take at home in pill form. He placed a call to my GP's office in Grapevine so that I could be sure to get in for additional medical treatment on Monday. He instructed me to take it easy and to put warm compresses on my breast for the next two days.

He drew with an ink pen around the red/pink lines on my breast. The infected area appeared to cover my entire right breast and extended even a little way up onto the left breast. The infected area also extended up under my right arm. He instructed Paul to watch to be sure that the red/pink area got smaller not larger. If the area got any larger, we were to return to the ER on Sunday.

We arrived home about eight, Saturday morning. Paul was nearly dead from exhaustion. Fighting this battle against Cancer had used up all of our stamina and strength. Paul always fought right beside me. Even though Paul was very tired from his overnight stint in the ER, he had to immediately leave our house after he got me into bed to go out to get my medicine and the bandaging things that I needed. While he was gone, I made calls to let everyone know that I would not be attending any more of the BeautiControl Seminar and that we would not be attending the wedding that afternoon. What a bummer!

After Paul got home with my medicine, I took my first doses, and we went to bed. Paul was just about "done in" from staying up all night, watching and waiting with me. I stayed in bed and rested after he got up that afternoon with hot compresses on my breast. I was taking big doses of the antibiotic.

More Lessons Learned

We learned more lessons that week. Even when I thought that things were okay, *I learned that I shouldn't ever really leave the area where my doctor was.* Earlier I had seen absolutely no reason why we should not have left Colorado to go to Texas when we did. However, I found out that there were many surprises that you can't predict that arise from nowhere when you have Cancer. The other thing that I guess I hadn't learned earlier with the pain management that I should have known was *to listen to my body.* If I had paid attention, I would have realized that my boob was going to bust. I should have reacted to this situation instead of passively just letting things happen. Who would have thought that I would spend the night in the emergency room with a burst breast? People wouldn't believe me if I had told this story in a crowd. They would have thought that I was just making a joke. *Cancer is not a disease for sissies!* One must be tough to fight Cancer!

Recovering Again

Life went on after the boob burst. I lay around the house all day Saturday using the dry heat on my breast. The heat helped to alleviate some of the pain. On Sunday morning to keep my routine as normal as possible, I put nursing pads into my bra to catch the bleeding from my new hole, and we went to church. After church, we went out to lunch with number 5 son and his family, John and Shelley Hyde and their children, Madeline and Gabby. Shelley's mother and father and her brother also came. I had missed one of the Daboub boy's wedding on Saturday that I had looked forward to attending. I enjoyed the big family gathering. Everyone pointed out that there was one good side to my Cancer—I had lost weight, and they could all see it. That was a good thing.

Life continued on as near to normal as we could make it. I attended a play, went to see my dentist, and packed to go to Houston. I also tried to reach my representative at MD Anderson to see if he could get me an appointment any earlier. I left several messages but never received a callback from him. The ER doctor had specifically told me to get in to see a surgeon right away. He had wanted me to see my regular family practice doctor on Monday. However, I didn't want to go in to see my family practice doctor because she had missed feeling my lump in my physical in December 2002. I was really mad at her for that. I didn't want to see a new surgeon in Grapevine when I was going to see a really good surgeon at MD Anderson on Thursday.

Paul and I watched my breast. The red streaks around the opening did decrease. I didn't seem to have any fever. My breast wound continued to drain, but by now, that seemed normal for me. I felt that I couldn't wait to get that awful breast removed. My right breast dripped blood continuously. My doctor daughter advised me to get nursing pads to wear inside my bras to keep the blood from ruining my clothes. These pads worked very well. My breast was finally beginning to feel a little better; however, the pain and soreness was still there. It was always tempting to try to exit out of this fight, to run away, and to never look back. I thought inside that maybe everything would be all right from now on all by itself. But I just couldn't quite give in to the temptation to stop the Cancer fight, although it was what I very much wanted to do.

Chapter 12

PATIENCE—FIGHTING CANCER IS NOT A RACE

The Trip to Houston

Wednesday, August 13, 2003, finally came, and we got in the car and drove to Houston. My breast was definitely better. The redness had gone down, but it was still swollen and hard. The open wound, where it had burst, still bled. My breast and underarm areas were still very sore. I was so glad to be heading to MD Anderson. I hoped that now we could finally get all of the Cancer out of my body and that I could begin the road to recovery. After all, MD Anderson was famous for its miracles and wonderful cures, at least this was what I hoped would happen for me. MD Anderson was a promise that I was counting on.

We planned to stay with Jeff and Liz Dittmer, our number one son and his wife, in Spring, Texas, a northern suburb in Houston. I hoped to soon have a plan from MD Anderson for my surgery to get this Cancer out of my body. In the meantime, I reminded myself that I had to keep working on another of the lessons that I was learning on my journey—*patience*. It always seemed to take so long to get anything accomplished.

I slept a lot on the drive to Houston that day. It is just about a four-hour drive from our house to our son's house in Spring. Jeff and Liz were always excellent hosts. They gave us our own room (the guest bedroom) when we stayed with them. It was nice to see Erica, our oldest granddaughter, again. She had grown that summer and would be twelve in September. She was getting to be quite a young lady. She was an extremely sweet grandchild to this old grandmother.

MD Anderson

A Reputable Cancer Hospital

MD Anderson is a medical institution that deals only with Cancer. It is full every day with people who have Cancer. People from all over the world come to Houston to be treated. Each one of them has Cancer. Every day there are thousands of people at this facility. A lot of the people come to MD Anderson only after they have depleted their local medical resources. MD Anderson turns no Texas resident away, and they take anyone from out of state that they can. They also treat lots of international patients from all over the world. They keep on staff a large supply of translators to help with the foreigners.

Since MD Anderson handles only Cancer, they have many specialized units that handle only a specific kind of Cancer. For example, I went to the Breast Clinic. My surgeon did nothing but breast surgeries all day long. My oncologists cared for only breast Cancer patients. MD Anderson always is running thousands of trials and studies to further research for Cancer treatments. They are one of the leading Cancer research facilities in the United States.

In 2003, when I went to Houston, MD Anderson and Sloan Kettering were probably ranked as the most prestigious Cancer facilities in the United States and probably the world. With all of this fame and specialty care, you may wonder why I didn't go to this hospital immediately.

What Took Me So Long to Get to MD Anderson

1. Ease.

It is important that you, my reader, understand my reasoning in this area so that you do not make the same mistakes that I made. The first reason that I didn't go to MD Anderson when I found the lump was because it was difficult. It was much easier to just live our life like we had been doing and to stay in our house and in our familiar surroundings. It was easier to be around my friends. It was easier to go to a local doctor in Durango. We had several nurse friends in Durango. Our good friend, Marge Rebovich, had worked with all of the doctors, especially the surgeons, in Durango over the many years of her career. She got me in to see the "best" and most-renowned surgeon there. It was just easier to stay in Durango.

2. It probably wasn't Cancer.

Second, whoever thinks that their lump is really Cancer? Why make an appointment at an out-of-state facility a "million miles" away when the odds are that it isn't Cancer anyway? Although I knew in my "heart of hearts" that my lump was Cancer, I never thought that I should bank on my feelings. Why make a big move when there was an 85 percent chance that the lump was benign?

    3.   Speed—Durango doctor could do next surgery quickly.

Even though it took me several weeks to have the surgery in Durango, I felt this was a much faster process than it would have been for me to figure out how to get to MD Anderson, make the trip there, and then to have the surgery 1,000 miles from our Durango home where we were living at the time. Although it seemed to take forever to get through the diagnosing and testing in Colorado, it seemed like it would be more efficient to do that work where we were rather than to pick up and go to Houston to do it.

You might ask, "Why didn't you go to MD Anderson after the first lumpectomy when you knew that you had Cancer?" I didn't go to MD Anderson right away because the Durango surgeon could do the second surgery quickly (only ten days after he had done the first lumpectomy). Looking back on the situation this is really the time that I should have gone. When we knew that I had Cancer, we should have packed our bags, closed the Colorado house, and gone immediately to Houston.

MD Anderson recommended at that time that you not have a lumpectomy immediately. They want the diagnosis of Cancer to be made with a biopsy, leaving the lump in place. They then preferred to use chemotherapy immediately to see if they can reduce the size of the lump before they remove the lump. By doing this, they can experiment and ascertain that they have the exact right recipe of chemicals (chemo formulas) that are good for fighting your particular Cancer. When I went to MD Anderson, my lump was nearly already gone. They used what their experience had led them to believe was the right chemical recipe to fight my Cancer in chemotherapy. I hope that they used a good "cocktail" and that my Cancer never returns.

I should have gone to MD Anderson immediately when I found out that I had Cancer. However, the doctor in Durango was really nice. In order to have gotten into MD Anderson, I probably would have used up a lot of time. As it turns out, I probably would not have wasted any time and might have actually saved time. However, one never knows what the future holds. Paul and I did what we thought was the best at the time. I am writing this book to help others make better decisions than I did.

When I was diagnosed with Cancer, my main objective and goal in life was to get that Cancer out of my body as quickly as I could. Nothing else seemed more important. However, I should have remembered that *the fight against Cancer is not a race.* I couldn't understand it, but I did not have to go so quickly in making my decisions and my moves. Getting rid of the monster Cancer was the most important thing to me, but I should have listened to others who told me not to rush. My results would have probably worked out just fine if I had slowed down and taken more time. However, my nature is to dive right in, and I had no intention of having Cancer one day longer than I absolutely had to. I made some mistakes and paid for this haste.

4. Lack of knowledge

I just didn't know enough about Cancer in general and its specific treatments to make the best judgments early in this game. I wasn't an expert on Breast Cancer in June or July of 2003. It took time and lots of help and experience for me to learn.

Keeping the First Appointment

Finding the Facility

On Thursday morning, I could hardly wait to get to MD Anderson. We followed the driving directions very carefully that the hospital staff had sent and got to the hospital without any trouble. It is scary driving in Houston. The freeways are big, crowded at all times of the day, and run really fast. We would learn our way around in the hospital district in time, but at this point, it was really an adventure just locating the big pink hospital building that was MD Anderson.

The MD Anderson Hospital is a *huge* place. I thought to myself as we drove up to this complex of buildings that lots of people must have Cancer. When we entered the main entrance, we were surrounded by people, some of whom looked very sick and fragile. There is a special look that people have when they are deep into the fight against Cancer. They often have no hair; they may wear a mask around their nose and mouth to keep germs away; their skin is translucent, very fragile, and pale-looking; and they are often in wheelchairs with an IV pole following them all around. Seeing all of these very sick people just fanned the flames of the fire of fear that burned in my belly. I worked each day to control this fire and to keep my life on the outside looking normal. It was really hard for me to see all of the strange people here at this big Cancer hospital and to think that soon I might look just like them.

Seeing the Doctor

We checked in without any problems and were directed to the Breast Center Clinic. There in a full waiting room, among about forty-five other patients, we sat and waited to be called. Our appointment was at 11:30 a.m. At 11:35 a.m. Dr. Ralston's nurse came out and told us that Dr. Ralston was running about fifteen to twenty-five minutes behind schedule. So we waited. However, the fifteen to twenty-five minutes turned into an hour and a half. We went back into an examining room about 1:00 p.m. It was hard for me to wait.

I was hoping that finally we could make positive plans to get rid of this Cancer. We first saw the nurse and Dr. Ralston's PA, Jori. I told both of these medical people that I had a breast that had burst. They all laughed at first. I know that they thought that I was joking, but their eyes got big when I pulled down my bra and they actually saw the open running sore. After the first look at my bare breast, they believed my strange tale. They didn't know immediately what to do about it, but at least they believed me. They left the room, and Paul and I sat alone.

Dr. Ralston finally came back into the examining room where Paul and I waited. He looked at my breast and explained that I had a hematoma. He asked if he could try to clear it some by mashing out the liquid. I said that he could, and I lay down. However, he didn't do anything but start to squeeze my breast, and I nearly jumped out of my skin. It hurt horribly. Quickly Dr. Ralston realized that he was hurting me. He immediately left the room with his entourage of students and Fellows. (MD Anderson is a teaching hospital, so you usually have accompanying associates with each doctor. Dr. Ralston is a professor in the University of Texas Medical School, located near MD Anderson, so he had a Resident and a Fellow accompanying him that day.)

He returned in just a few minutes later, apologizing profusely for having hurt me. He then asked me if I would like to get this thing fixed. I told him emphatically that I would like that very much. I suggested that he might just want to take the complete breast off because I was really tired of it. This request completely startled him. He answered me very seriously, saying that he could not take the breast off with all of the infection that I had. He just refused to do that. He said that I would have to go to another doctor if I wanted to get a mastectomy at this time. Well, this kind of set me back, but I quickly regrouped and told him that I would do as he felt I should. He explained that he would go into the open area and clean everything out so that the infection could completely heal. After about thirty days if the infection was gone, he then would schedule a mastectomy for me if that was what I wanted.

After we had agreed upon this course of action, he said that he would be finished with his clinic appointments at six that afternoon and that if I hurried, I could get the necessary tests run so that I could have the clean-out surgery done that evening. Fortunately, I had not eaten any lunch. He put me on a no-liquid and no-food diet retroactively, and we set off to get things done. Dr. Ralston said that he would go into my right breast surgically and remove the hematoma. I thought that this would make me better, so I was happy.

Chapter 13

THE JOURNEY CAN BE FULL OF UNEXPECTED TURNS—JUST GO ON

Preparing for Clean-out Surgery

It seemed a bit strange just walking into this big hospital and finding out that I would immediately have surgery. We had not brought anything with us. I had nothing—no toothbrush, no gown, no house shoes, not even my skin care or makeup. Paul had to do some calling to let Jeff and Liz know that we would not return to their house that evening as expected. He also needed to share this new plan with our family and called some of our other children.

After all of the hospital questions and forms about the immediate surgery had been completed, I felt ready. Someone was going to fix this hole in my breast that had been such a problem. The afternoon passed very quickly. We did a lot of walking in getting ourselves around to the many different departments in this large facility in order to do the testing and labwork that was called for before I could have the surgery. Fortunately, everyone at MD Anderson is very helpful about giving directions, and we were able to find our way in this huge maze.

Soon I was lying on the hospital gurney, getting prepped for surgery, and the nurse was checking all my tests and records. It was just about 6:00 p.m., and I surely wanted to be ready when Dr. Ralston arrived. The nurse checked everything and then asked if I had gotten an EKG that afternoon. I had not. She said, "Oh, no. We must have an EKG before we do this surgery." I thought just a minute and remembered that I had undergone an EKG in Durango before my second lumpectomy just a few weeks ago. I had the record of this EKG in my medical notebook, which we had with us in a cloth-carrying bag. I told the nurse. I got my medical book from Paul, who had the big job of carrying this notebook with us, and I turned through the tabs to my EKG section. I pulled out the recent EKG lab test results and handed it to the nurse. She checked it over and reported that this was wonderful. She went off, made a copy of this record, and inserted it into my file. I put the original back into my notebook, and I was ready for my surgery.

Keeping meticulous medical records from doctors, tests, hospital stays, etc., and carrying them with me had definitely paid off this day. You just never know when this big book would be needed. I still keep this book. It is now in two 3-inch binders that are stuffed full. However, the books are often useful.

Third Surgery

Quickly I went off to sleep for my third surgery before I even saw Dr. Ralston again. Surgery dates, so far, on this unplanned journey had been July 11 and 21 and now August 14. In just over a month, I had undergone three surgeries. On one hand, I wanted things to move quickly so that I could get through this ordeal that had taken over my life. However, my body was having a hard time keeping up and healing as I hurried along my path. Looking back on things now, I can see why living and recovering had been so hard. No wonder I was having a little trouble keeping things together.

Anyway, I woke up about 9:30 p.m. in the recovery room. I couldn't talk. My throat hurt this time from the inside because of the tube that is usually inserted in the throat during surgeries. I had a nurse that was assigned to just me and one other patient. She was busy doing the things that recovery nurses do. At about 11:30 p.m., I probably should have been sent up to a hospital room. However, there were no rooms available, so they decided that I would simply stay in the recovery room until a room became available the following day. I wondered what my insurance would think about that. Paul left to go home to Jeff's house to sleep a while after it was decided that I was going to stay in the recovery room.

Recovery Room Trial

I took pain shots through my IV and floated. I woke up every half hour because the lights were always on. In this experience, I think that I found out how the prisoners who are kept in brightly lighted cells must feel. There was activity, and people were all around all of the time. There was always someone walking about, and there was talking and noise. It was not a good place for sleeping. People were moaning and almost crying. I was fairly comfortable, but it seemed like the night lasted *forever*. It was the longest night that I had spent in ages. It seemed even longer than the night that I had spent in the Grapevine ER.

Paul had told me that he would come back early the next morning so that he could be present when the doctor came. I kept looking for him every time I woke up. 6:00 a.m. eventually arrived and so did Paul. I had been in an anesthetic stupor all night, and I just didn't like that. I was very glad to see Paul. Now that he had arrived, I knew that he would take care of things. I could relax again. Paul couldn't stay with me in the recovery room, but he could come back to see me regularly.

I continued to get the pain shots, and I even got up to go to the bathroom. A bit of normalcy really came back when I ate a little breakfast. I am sure that they do not normally serve meals in the surgical recovery room, but they did this day. I now had on a new bra, a compression bra that held my bandages all in place without any tape. My breast was still leaking, but now it looked more like dirty water instead of dark, red blood. In fact, on Friday morning my breast leaked so much that it went through my bandages and got my bra and my gown dirty. I explained to my nurse that I was accustomed to this and that my bandage needed checking and changing every few hours. I don't think that she liked my advice, but she changed everything and fixed me up good as new. The recovery room nurses were very good.

Healing at MD Anderson Hospital

At about 10:30 a.m., I was finally assigned my own room. My nurse packed me up, and one of the MD Anderson traveling folks pushed my bed, my things, and me to my new room. I didn't have to do a thing. I didn't even have to get from one bed to another. They settled the bed that I was on and me into the new room. It was tiny with only one chair and a TV. I had a small bathroom and a window that looked out on the other side of a building. I had a number to call to order my meals. I would order from a restaurant-like menu. I had a number to call if my room was too hot or too cold. I had a nurse and an assistant who were assigned to take care of me. I had call buttons on both sides of my bed and on a control from the wall. It seemed to be a very nice and safe hospital room.

I spent most of the afternoon waiting to get a sonogram scan of my left breast and the lymph nodes under my left arm. The scan came back negative. It appeared that I had no Cancer in my left breast or in any adjacent lymph nodes on that side. This was good news. The way this journey had been going, I was ready for a little good news.

I felt that I was finally moving down the road toward getting rid of this Cancer and in defining the exact Cancer battle that I had to fight. MD Anderson seemed to hold the key to unlocking the doors to reveal my future path. With this first bit of good news, I was feeling that a small ray of hope had somehow filtered through the clouds of fear and doubt that covered my being.

What Was My Clean-out Surgery

On Saturday morning, my surgeon's resident came by, and I was able to find out what had been done to my breast. Dr. Ralston had opened up my breast and had taken out over three cups of blood and infection fluids. He had cleaned out the site where the two earlier lumpectomies had been performed. He had cauterized a few blood vessels, and had packed the clean area with five yards of gauze tape. A little piece of this gauze hung out in the opening at the side of the wound just below my nipple. I now had an open cavity and an open entrance to this hematoma area.

The doctor explained that the gauze packing had to be changed daily. All you had to do to change this gauze was to get a good hold of the piece of gauze that was sticking out of my breast and slowly pull it all out. Then you got a new long strip of clean gauze tape and wet all of it with sterile saline solution. Then you needed to poke this clean wet gauze back into the cavity until you filled it up. The doctor did the first change as he was talking. Amazingly, this changing didn't hurt too badly. It looked and sounded a lot worse than it felt. The doctor told me that Paul should prepare to do this packing. Upon hearing this announcement, Paul and I both nearly died and indicated that we didn't think that we could do this. The doctor looked a little perplexed but said that we could get home health services to do it for us then. Another lesson in my Cancer walk learnings—*be prepared to submit to and perform all kinds of medical procedures.*

Our reluctance or fear of performing these daily gauze changes had not been in our doctor's plan. He had planned on releasing me very soon. However, the doctor wanted to keep me on an intravenous drip, or IV, to combat the infections that I had, so the hospital seemed the logical place for me to stay for a few days. This gave us more time to prepare ourselves for the tasks that lay ahead of us (daily gauze changing).

Hospital Boredom

After the excitement of the morning with the daily chores and the doctor's visit was over, my room became very quiet. Lying in a hospital bed has never been my idea of fun. I began to think that maybe some people died of boredom in the hospital. I had caught up on my lost sleep Friday afternoon and night. I didn't really have the energy to get up and walk around everywhere, but it really was tough staying in my room all day.

Fortunately, Liz and Erica came to see me not too long after the doctor left. They brought several games, which promised to brighten my idle time. Peter, Sondra, Fritz, Foster, and Grant (number two son and his family) also arrived to visit. I received a gorgeous rose flower arrangement from John (number five son) and his wife and girls. The arrangement had a white teddy bear attached, and the sweet card pointed out that Madeline and Gabby (their children—two sweet grandchildren) had insisted upon sending these flowers that had the bear. They knew that I liked stuffed animals and that I would enjoy this special "teddy" from them.

At lunchtime, all of my visitors went down to the cafeteria to eat. My small room would not accommodate everyone. However, I was most thankful for the visitors and the distractions they provided from my hospital boredom. Everyone left by two that afternoon. I was tired and slept for a couple of hours. I still didn't feel good and promptly threw up my lunch. I had switched today from the drip IV antibiotic to the horse-pill form of the same medicine, which can cause you to be nauseated. The nurse brought in an antinausea drip bag for my supper. I was ready to stay in my bed and rest.

I must tell you about the hospital bed that I had. You program it with your weight, and then as you move on the bed, it automatically fluffs itself up around your pressure points. It takes all the strains and pressures off of your body when you lay in the bed. It was the most comfortable hospital bed that I had ever been in. It stayed with me all through my hospital stay and was fabulous. I wish that I could have brought it home with me.

The hospital resident doctor for Dr. Ralston changed the gauze in my breast wound daily. Paul and I still worried about what we were going to do about changing it when I left the hospital.

Going Home in Houston to Heal

A Restful Sunday

Sunday morning, August 17, about eleven, I left MD Anderson Hospital and went home with Paul to recuperate at Jeff's house. I had gone into the hospital on Thursday night. My stay had been short. I rested in bed that Sunday afternoon in my home away from home. My pain level was very low now, but I was weak. It was nice to be around family in a home environment.

The doctor had changed the gauze in my breast that morning before we left the hospital, so we had a little more time before we needed to perform this brand-new procedure. The open wound had to be repacked every day. We were planning to go to MD Anderson each day to get this done. How was this going to work?

Monday—A Test Day

Monday, we had to go to MD Anderson anyway because I had appointments for two more tests to help the doctors determine if the Cancer had metastasized to any other part of my body. The first test was a bone scan, and it was easy. They put an IV in my arm and injected me with radioisotopes. They then had me wait an hour for these isotopes to get into my bones. They next put me on a metal table and told me to lie really still for ten minutes as the big machine ran over my body. The technician had to run the machine a second time because the area under my right breast was all solid. He had me lay over on my side for a second scan. I didn't hear the results of this test until we met with the doctor on Thursday of that week.

Immediately following the bone scan, I went into another area and underwent a CT scan. I was required to drink thirty-six fluid ounces of flavored barium. It was cold and thick and not very appetizing, but I drank it.

The lab was still full of people even though it was 4:00 p.m. You could tell who the patients were because all of us were sitting around with big white cups of flavored barium in our hands. Each patient had at least one caregiver or support person with him. Some people had three or four people waiting with them. By the end of the day, I was tired and worn out.

Drinking thirty-six fluid ounces of chalky-tasting stuff was not fun, but I guessed that it was necessary. I drank the last twelve ounces, changed into a hospital gown, and was taken into the scan room. There I lay again on a metal table/bed. For this scan, I had a round machine over me that talked and instructed me to breathe in, to breathe out, and to hold my breath. The nurse injected a shot of iodine into my veins through the IV that was still in my arm from the earlier scan. The iodine gave me a real heat rush. My whole body felt like it got hot from the inside out. Then the round machine moved over my body. Quickly this test was over, and I was done. The nurse removed my IV, and I put my clothes back on. I had only had two tests, but it had taken all day. Everything seemed to take a long time at MD Anderson.

This had been a busy and not too difficult day, except that we hadn't had time to get my breast repacked. We went back up to the Breast Clinic. Even though it was after 5:30 p.m., the Breast Clinic was still working. They had an on-call nurse who handles the kinds of things like packing my breast in the clinic each day. She changed the gauze in my breast, and we were finally finished at MD Anderson for that day. It was after 7:30 p.m. when we got to Sondra and Peter's, our number two son's house. I was exhausted and went immediately to bed. Paul had to handle all of the social amenities that evening.

Peter and Sondra live in Friendswood, which is a suburb on the south side of Houston, just past NASA. It is an hour's drive between Jeff's house in Spring and Peter's house in Friendswood. MD Anderson is just about in the middle between the two houses. We were very fortunate to have two children living in this area. We were never required to stay in a motel while we were treating this Cancer in Houston.

Tuesday, Going Back Just to Get the Gauze Changed

We went back to MD Anderson on Tuesday only to have the gauze changed in my breast. It took us nearly an hour to drive there and then another two hours to meet the nurse and to get the change made. We decided that it was time that Paul learned how to do the gauze change. The nurse that we saw that Tuesday helped Paul with instructions and then prepared a list of materials that we would need at home. We went down to the dispensary, turned in our needed supply list, and waited until our order was filled.

We walked out with a big white shopping bag full of saline solution, big swab sticks (used to poke the gauze in), yards and yards of clean gauze, big gauze pads to make bandages, and tape. With these supplies, we thought that we were prepared to perform the gauze changes ourselves. Paul would do the changing, and I would allow him to do it. Paul's mother had been a surgical nurse, so he grew up under the tutelage of a medical caregiver. He had no qualms or fears of being able to do the change out. I, however, was a little bit afraid to have Paul doing this, but I surely didn't like spending half a day at MD Anderson each day either.

I was beginning to really start to feel better. My breast finally seemed to be getting well. The redness around my wound was nearly all gone. The swelling and the extreme soreness had

Chapter 14

THE DECISION-MAKING COMMITTEE IS A NECESSITY

My Medical Decision Committee

Before we left Colorado, Paul and I discovered that we were getting medical advice from everyone. Everyone loved us and meant well. However, everyone's knowledge and experience was different and was sometimes very lacking. As we made the decision to move my treatment to MD Anderson, we also made the decision that we should set up a medical decision committee for me. The committee would be made up of the people with the most knowledge and love for me. The committee would have three members so that there would never be a tie or a time of indecision. The members would be me, Paul, and my doctor daughter, Mary Joy.

Paul is my husband of nearly twenty years and loved me very much. Mary Joy is an ob-gyn doctor and is not a Cancer specialist, but she worked in a hospital with Cancer specialists whom she consulted frequently. She was also well equipped to do her own research on medical issues, and she often did the research that she felt was necessary. She was a wonderful help and source of factual information.

I really would recommend to anyone who has to journey down this road that you set up a decision committee similar to this. You receive medical advice from lots of people each day. These people are very loving and caring people. However, they are just not in the best position to make your medical decisions. You are also asked to make decisions by doctors. Sometimes different doctors recommend different things. You and your medical committee have to sort through the counseling and make these decisions together.

At the beginning of this journey, I was confused. I kind of muddled around and made mistakes. I didn't really know what I should be doing when. When I realized that I was bungling this job and needed a formal method, Paul and I thought that by establishing a formal process, we could make wiser choices. Mary Joy was very willing to become an active part of this

BREAST CANCER: THE UNPLANNED JOURNEY - LESSONS LEARNED

all but disappeared. Maybe I could get back to a normal life sometime in the near future. I had hopes of returning to our home, our family, and our friends in Grapevine.

Later in the Week at MD Anderson

MD Anderson is an effective, efficient, huge Cancer-fighting facility. The place appeared to be overcrowded, but everyone eventually got served and cared for. No one asked us to pay a penny up front. No one even talked about money or payments. It was hard to find our way around this giant facility, but we were learning. It wasn't easy to drive in Houston, but we were learning our way there also. Paul, my husband, was my constant and never-failing companion. I truly don't know what I would have done without him. He sat patiently waiting all day in the waiting rooms that were full of Cancer patients. He read and sat quietly, constantly trying to help me in any way that he could.

I still cried a lot. Having the strength to endure the pokings, the probings, and the tests each day was difficult. Thinking of the way that this disease attacks a body, retires, and then attacks somewhere else was really scary. I learned by seeing all of the thousands of Cancer patients at MD Anderson that *only the positive, tough people survive Cancer.*

Being surrounded all day by people who may be dying of Cancer was difficult for me. Only on Thursday, August 21, when I went back to my doctor and got the results of the many tests that I had undergone, did I find out that I might be different from them. I found out that there is a good chance that I will beat this disease and will live a long and normal life. This news made my day and gave me fuel to fight off the Cancer monster that roared in my inner being!

committee. We just didn't tell the rest of the family what was going on. After establishing our decision-making procedures, I was able to listen lovingly to all of the advice that was given me without being confused or overwhelmed. I knew that the actual decision would be made by my medical committee. Making medical decisions through this committee helped me a lot.

Another Lumpectomy or a Mastectomy?

When Paul and I went in to talk to my surgeon, Dr. Ralston on August 21, we were asked if I wanted another lumpectomy. This was the first decision that my medical committee had to make. I was very tired and weary of surgeries and didn't really want more. However, my medical committee, Mary Joy, Paul, and I discussed this situation at length. Using her research and knowledge, Mary Joy explained to Paul and me that the kind of Cancer that I had, lobular filtrating carcinoma, would come back to my breasts even if at this point in time they surgically removed all of it from my body. She said that I should *not* even attempt to have another lumpectomy. She even went as far as to say that the odds were very high that I would get this Cancer in my left breast in the future. She highly recommended that I get a double mastectomy.

A Single or a Double Mastectomy?

As the time (September 15, 2003, when my breast surgery was scheduled) drew near, we had to decide whether I was going to have a single or a double mastectomy. All of the tests at MD Anderson had been run, and it looked like my left breast was clear of any Cancer. The surgeon would do exactly what I wanted in this matter without making any recommendations to us. I had already had so much surgery and complications that I wanted to have a simple single mastectomy on the right breast. I was just tired of hurting and of being sick. However, my doctor daughter, Mary Joy, and Paul both thought that I should have a double mastectomy. I wanted the single mastectomy because of the pain involved. I was getting to be a real sissy about surgeries. In making my decision, I was only looking at the immediate future. Paul and especially Mary Joy were looking at the long term prospects for my life.

Mary Joy gave us two reasons for recommending that I have a double mastectomy. She pointed out that since I had lobular carcinoma infiltrating Cancer and my left breast surely had lobular carcinoma in situ all in it, at some time down the road (five, ten, or even twenty years), I would get Cancer in the left breast. She secondly indicated that my body would forever be off balanced with one large left breast and no right breast. I would be forced to always wear a heavy prosthesis. I really did not want the hurt, the pain, and the complications of having a double mastectomy. I just didn't want to go through another big surgery. However, my vote was the only one against the double mastectomy.

Paul, after listening to Mary Joy, thought that I definitely should have the double mastectomy. So the decision was made. I was overruled, but I wasn't unhappy. In a loving effort to make me feel better, Mary Joy pointed out that I would not have to worry about the Cancer coming back in my left breast and that was a relief for me. My medical committee outvoted me on this issue and decided that I should have the double mastectomy rather than another lumpectomy or a single mastectomy (which I favored). I trusted the medical committee that we had set up. I very much trusted my lovely daughter's judgments just as she had trusted mine when she was growing up. This turned out to be one of the wisest decisions that was made during the unplanned journey.

Chapter 15

KEEP REMINDERS OF LOVE AND SUPPORT WITH YOU

My Yellow Comfort Bag

When you are going through the stresses of hospital tests, surgeries, and treatments, you need to be prepared to lean on the mementos of support and love that you have received from others. I found that I wanted to be able to put my hands around that hard, smooth, cool comfort stone to remember my new friend who had also gone through breast Cancer. I felt that feeling close to her through holding this stone would make me stronger and more able to endure my trials.

You need to be able to read some of the loving writings that you have received in "get well" cards from your friends and family. Prepare a bag in which you can carry some of these items with you when you go to the clinic and the hospital. You never know when it is going to be an especially tough day, and you may need a mental "pick me up," which you can get from reading again the card that your best friend sent when she heard that you had Cancer. I never knew when the pain might get to be intolerable for a few moments in a test and how comforting it would be to hold that soft fluffy teddy bear that two of my grandchildren sent to me.

I had found a lovely yellow canvas bag that was decorated with bows. The bows were made of three-fourth-inch brograin ribbon, and each one was a different bright basic color. The bag was bright and sunny. I decided while we were still in Colorado to put my special things into this bag so that I could carry them with me when I went to the hospital for treatments. The bag grew heavier as the days passed, and I received more tokens of encouragement from my dear friends. The bag carried a little love from each of my supporters, and I would draw from their strength and encouragement when I most needed it as I walked the unplanned journey.

The Special Heart Pillow

Another one of my strengthening momentos was a small pillow that was made in the shape of a heart. When I walked into MD Anderson the first time, I met the MD Anderson volunteers. They helped us immediately when we entered the front door of this big hospital. In the Breast Clinic, the volunteers had a table set up that contained cookies and candy, pink ribbons, and information about breast Cancer and MD Anderson events. Their table was near the check-in area. After I had finished my check-in form-filling-out routine, one of the volunteers greeted me, and I went over to their table. There were two nicely dressed women standing behind their table. They introduced themselves, and I found that they had each fought breast Cancer. All of the volunteers at MD Anderson are Cancer survivors, so they knew firsthand what the patients were going through.

These ladies wanted to help in any way that they could. When they found out that I was a new breast Cancer patient at MD Anderson, they gave me a ten-inch soft heart-shaped pillow. The lady told me to put this pillow under my arm when I sat or slept. She explained that it cushioned the sore areas. She also said that this pillow was handmade by a loving lady for me. I took the pink flowered-print pillow and thanked the ladies for being such a help.

Everywhere that I went in this hospital, I saw the MD Anderson volunteers. When you had to spend hours waiting for doctors, for tests, and for nurses, they would come around to offer conversation, candy, and a word of encouragement. They ran a refreshment cart that they drove through the entire hospital in the morning and then again in the afternoon that contained coffee, tea, cokes, muffins, cup cakes, candy, cookies, and fruit that you could purchase. We often had to wait long periods of time, and the volunteers refreshment cart was a welcome interruption in those long times. The volunteers were very helpful, warm, comforting, and encouraging. I kept my little pillow with me until my surgical wounds were all healed.

Chapter 16

Good News along the Journey!—Seeing a Light at the End of the Unplanned Journey

After-Surgery Checkup

Test Results

We made our "sum it up" visit after my clean-out surgery to MD Anderson on Thursday, August 21. We met again with my surgeon, Dr. Kimble Ralston, and his associate. The open hematoma wound that Dr. Ralston had cleaned out looked good. His instructions were for us to keep on changing the gauze each day. He said that hopefully, in a month, the wound would heal completely from the inside and would not hold any gauze at all. We could already tell that the length of gauze that Paul was able to poke in each day was getting shorter. Remember we started by poking in five yards of gauze.

My CT scan showed that everything was normal with my organs. The bone scan showed that the Cancer had not metastasized to my bones. All of this was very good. This made my Cancer a T2, N1 Cancer or a stage 2 Cancer. This meant that the chance of it reoccurring in my body was 40 percent. However, after chemotherapy, the chance of the Cancer reoccurring would be cut to 20 percent. This was good news.

Double Mastectomy Plans

Dr. Ralston asked me what we had decided to do. I told him that I wanted a double mastectomy and that I did not want reconstruction. With this information, he estimated that I would be in the hospital for two nights. He indicated that we could leave Houston when I left the hospital after the mastectomies. Neither Paul nor I wanted to leave the MD Anderson area that soon. I would have drains from each of the mastectomies. These drains would have to stay in for approximately two weeks. I asked about the recovery time (I meant time when I was free from painkillers) from this surgery, and Dr. Ralston replied that recovery time should be about the same time as when the drains came out. He indicated that when the drains came out, I should be nearly pain free again.

We questioned whether I would need radiation therapy or not. He indicated that my case was on the border and that they would make that decision after my surgery. There was a clinical trial going on now that I would be eligible for (if they found no more Cancer with my next surgery). This trial was examining whether it was better to have radiation therapy or not to have it for the long prognosis.

Dr. Ralston would be on vacation the first part of September. He would do my surgery on Monday, September 15. He checked my current hematoma breast again and reported that everything looked good. Because I had had infection already in this breast, the chances of problems and infections with the mastectomy were increased. Dr. Ralston thought that we would still probably have a wick sticking out at this time (in other words, it would not have completely closed and healed). He indicated that right now, everything looked good. He said that there was very little Cancer left in that breast and that our waiting to do the mastectomy would have no effect on my long-term survival prognosis. Dr. Ralston left the details of the surgery to be handled by his assistant, and went on back to his busy schedule and other patients.

His assistant set about to tell me about the planned surgery. I signed the consent forms. They would do a right modified mastectomy. They would go back in and look for any more lymph nodes under the right arm and in the breast area. They would take out any lymph nodes that they found on the right side because these nodes had already showed that they were infected with Cancer. They would do a sentinel node biopsy on the left breast. They would find the sentinel nodes and would do frozen biopsies on each one. If they found any nodes through the biopsies with Cancer in them, they would remove the sentinel nodes and the lymph nodes behind them on the left side. If they did not find Cancer in any of the sentinel nodes, they would reserve the right after a better biopsy could be performed (after a few days) to go back in to remove the nodes if any Cancer was found. A frozen biopsy is only 85 percent accurate. If there was Cancer in the left side lymph nodes, they would then do a modified mastectomy on the left breast.

My Feelings about the Planned Surgery

I did so hope that there was no Cancer anywhere on the left side of my body, especially not in the lymph nodes. Removing lymph nodes and cutting through those arm and shoulder muscles seemed to be more painful than breast surgery. My arm cuts had certainly been more painful than the breast cut after my second lumpectomy. I hoped that I could keep my left arm healthy and with its lymph nodes. I still slept and sat with my special heart Cancer pillow under my right arm. The softness and cushioning of the pillow helped to keep the pain level down.

I did not look forward to another major surgery. However, I knew that to beat this Cancer, surgery was the best way to immediately get it out of my body. I was just now beginning to feel healthy again from my three earlier surgeries. It seemed that I had been sick and completely weighted down with this disease since it was diagnosed with the first lumpectomy on July 11. I think that my decisions were now colored by "how much pain would be involved" rather than on what each procedure actually gave me and the best long-term prognosis.

I was forced to trust my medical advisors, my daughter, Mary Joy, and my husband, Paul, more as we got farther along this road, and I became more weighted down with the battle against the disease. I was becoming weary and might not be as clear and analytical as I had been before I began this journey. I very much trusted the knowledge and the abilities of my two chief advisors though, so I was okay. My support system seemed to be in place.

The Unplanned Journey Education Continued

I knew that I would be required to go through chemotherapy. Dr. Ralston indicated that if I did not do radiation therapy the chemotherapy would start two to three weeks after my surgery. Chemotherapy generally lasted for six months. Radiation therapy normally lasted for six weeks. This all meant that I would be finished with my treatments by June of next year. I immediately took June as the goal for my completion date of the unplanned journey.

I knew that Paul and I were going to want very badly to return to Colorado next summer, and I was happy to know that the doctors thought that we might be able to. I wanted to start living again. I wanted to get into shape to climb some of those beautiful Colorado mountains. Walking the unplanned journey kept us focused on Cancer. We had no time, energy, or resources to indulge in the pleasures that we had so freely enjoyed before Cancer hit. It was good to know that the unplanned journey might have an end to it!

We were ecstatic about the Cancer evaluation report that we had received from Dr. Ralston What a relief! He had actually quantified with statistics the different Cancer situations. He had staged my Cancer as a T2, N1. The testing that MD Anderson had done made him confident in saying that at this time, I had no other Cancers growing in my body. Up until this time, no one had been able to give us this kind of information. Not knowing what I was facing or the extent to which the Cancer had invaded my body was very difficult. We now could say that my long-term forecast was good. I might actually live a long and useful life after all. We had facts and information, and the information was good!

I had spent several months recognizing that I had Cancer. I had endured numerous invasive and unpleasant tests and surgeries. I had suffered physical pain. I had realized that death was a real and looming possible outcome. I had seen the death shadow reflected in the eyes of my friends and family as they recognized the seriousness of my diagnosis. All of these experiences left me very humbled. Realizing that I was weak and that I did not control my own destiny or the way that my life might go was difficult for me. Spending even only a week at MD Anderson was an education in itself on the unplanned journey. And I didn't know it but there were many more things ahead for me to learn.

Chapter 17

THE DARKEST TIME

It was sometime during this restful, getting-well time that my mind's worries got out of hand. Somehow deep in my soul I felt that I was going to die in the mastectomy surgery or shortly thereafter. I did not think that I would have another time of health and happiness. Actually I was in a time of rest and waiting. I couldn't have the mastectomy until September 15. I didn't really feel bad. I had to see that my gauze stuffing and bandages were changed each day, but I was definitely on the mend. It was only late August. I like to refer to this as my time of sabbatical away from surgery and the actual day-to-day battle against Cancer.

Because I thought that I might never live a productive and happy life again, I set about with another mission—I needed to see everyone that I loved. I needed to have them see me as happy and controlled. I had been such a crying wimp during the first part of this Cancer battle that I was ashamed. I didn't want any of my family and my friends to remember me that way. I wanted their last thoughts of me to be happy ones. So I set about to see everyone one more time.

I wrote the following in my writings at the time:

> Paul is busy working getting chores and tasks done around the house. I am not taking on these jobs. I have gone back to the daily housekeeping chores, but I am letting him handle all the big stuff. I am on sabbatical from my Cancer battle, and I am resting and "making hay while the sun shines." Since I never know what lies ahead with this disease, I must do the important things while I have the strength and the energy.

This is as close as I ever came to putting into words the secret fears that I had of dying. I thought that my life if I lived would never be the same again and would forever be horribly different. I don't know even today exactly what I thought, but inside I was very, very scared. On the outside I expressed confidence. In fact, I boasted of beating the Cancer completely in my newsletter. Read the following from my newsletter dated August 8, 2003:

I, with God's, Paul's, Mary Joy's, the doctors', my friends', and my family's help, will beat this Cancer so badly that it will not return to eat away at my strength and my body. It invaded me quietly and lay growing and dormant for many years. But I know it's there now, and I will beat it and destroy it. The battle is on!

My emotions were bouncing everywhere. To the outside world, I was confident and assured. I very much wanted to portray this "perfect and in control" visage, but inside I was eaten up with fear. The fires of doubt, uncertainty, pain, and terror nearly consumed my soul at this time.

However, my saga continued as I traveled down the road of this unplanned journey. I discovered another lesson. I realized that the old saying—*It gets darkest just before the dawn*—was true at least in my life. You have to get all of the bad news; you have to get completely to the bottom of the hole before you can begin to climb out again. Getting to the bottom was hard. I thought that I had now bottomed out and was on my way to make the climb out. I asked my supporters to keep on pulling for me so that I could make it. I knew that it would not be an easy climb out. I already knew that *Cancer was not a disease that I could beat by myself. I needed help*. I worked very hard at keeping the death monster quieted inside of me, and I waited.

Chapter 18

USE ALL RESOURCES

Returning to MD Anderson

On Wednesday, September 3, Paul and I traveled back to Houston to have my breast wound checked. While waiting in the Breast Center area, we found a brochure advertising an interesting seminar entitled "The Unplanned Journey—Living Fully with Cancer." The seminar was scheduled for that very weekend in Houston.

My breast exam checked out fine. On Thursday morning, we finished our work at MD Anderson. We completed all of our pre-op procedures and papers, and I finished the morning's work by getting copies of my records for my medical notebook.

"The Unplanned Journey—Living Fully with Cancer"

We were now free to spend the rest of my sabbatical time as we wanted. Paul and I talked about the seminar. It looked like they were going to have some famous people speaking. We wondered at this late date (the seminar started that afternoon) if there would even be space for two more attendees, but having nothing to really loose, we called the registration number from MD Anderson. As it turns out, they were still taking registrations. We decided to go. This turned out to be one of the most valuable things that we did. This seminar gave me the opportunity to become acquainted with a lot of people who were successfully battling Cancer. I highly recommend to anyone that travels this same road *study how other people have successfully beaten Cancer.* This is a way of arming yourself and gathering your fighting equipment for the Cancer battle that you face.

On Thursday afternoon, we went to this seminar. The MD Anderson Network was the sponsoring organization. This network solicited contributions so that the cost for the conference participant was very low, only $60. (We ate $60 worth of food at dinners and banquets while we were there). The conference attendance fee was the biggest bargain that I had seen in a long time.

All of the Cancer drug manufacturers were there with their brochures and information. There were about 650 Cancer patients, survivors, and their caregivers attending.

Some of the speakers included, Dr. Bob Arnot, Ted Kennedy Jr., and Dr. John Mendelsohn (the president of MD Anderson). Their talks were magnificent and inspiring. The seminar included wellness workshops on Tai Chi, journaling, rest and relaxation, taming your inner dragons, relaxation messages, Tibetan meditation, and yoga. We heard lots of very interesting speeches. Some of the topics covered were "New Advances in the Treatment of Cancer," "Facing the Challenge," "Don't Look Back—We're Not Going that Way," and "Survive to Win."

We enjoyed listening to panels of doctors and of Cancer survivors. We learned tons of new things about Cancer and its treatments. Paul and I found that it was impossible to participate in all of the offerings. We were forced to choose which breakout sessions we wanted to attend. We felt that if we split up, we could absorb more materials and information, so each of us went our separate ways with notepads in hand for luncheons, breakout sessions, and other separately held meetings. Each of us was obligated to share the information that we learned with the other one.

Breakout Session "Rest and Relaxation"— Inner Mind Symbols Reflect Your Life

The first breakout session that I went to was on "rest and relaxation." The instructor guided us through a "close your eyes and take deep breaths" routine that I had seen before. I participated under her guidance and did feel better when the routine was over. I didn't know yet if I had enough discipline to actually use this technique on myself. At the end of the session, I promised that I would certainly try to use this technique when I needed it, however. In fighting my Cancer battle, I wanted all of the ammunition that I could gather.

Next, the instructor gave each of us paper and colors and asked us to draw our internal private gardens that we had finally gone to in the "close your eyes" routine that I just described. I, of course, drew my garden so that it contained tall, pointed rocky mountains, pine trees, red flowers, a deer, a cat, and a river with rocks in it. I drew a bright sun, and on the left-hand side, near the top of the paper, I drew a big rock with a black monster on it just below the sun. The monster had many legs and arms and hair that fuzzed all over his head. My drawing looked like a child's picture. My figures were not beautiful, nor did my trees look like real pine trees. My cat and my deer at least were very identifiable, however, and the rocks were dark with only simple detail. However, I quickly discerned that the teacher was not trying to make us artists. She wanted us to try to communicate what was inside our minds. She wanted us to open up and to share our hidden thoughts and fears.

After we had taken a few minutes to complete our drawings, the teacher went around to each of us and talked about our works individually. When the teacher analyzed my picture, she immediately started talking about my red flowers. She pointed out that they were not well rooted and that red was the color of blood and fire. She saw the river and counted the rocks that I had drawn in it. I had unconsciously drawn seven stones in the river. She counted them and then asked me what month I had been diagnosed with Cancer. Of course, I was diagnosed in July, the seventh month of the year.

Her analysis of my picture was interesting, and now I think of my internal private garden as looking just like my life's picture. I had already experienced blood in the surgeries and the wounds that I had. I was happy to find also that my flowers didn't appear to be well rooted. I thought that this probably showed that I wasn't looking for too much more blood ahead of me. The fact that my garden was in Colorado probably meant that I longed to get back there to happy times again.

I knew that I had to slay the monster (Cancer). The monster would stay a threat and a ruination of the peace in my beautiful garden (in my life) until somehow it was destroyed. I hoped that before another few years passed, my life would be free of Cancer and then my internal garden would not have a monster in it. My drawing of that day was not a picture that I ever wanted to frame, but it was one that I keep to remind me of *my inner mind symbols* and how they *reflected my life* and my fears at that time.

Breakout Session "Journaling"— Communicate Your Inner Fears and Feelings

The second session that I attended that afternoon was on journaling, taught by Sandi Stromberg, MA. Mrs. Stromberg talked a moment about her journaling and then read us a poem entitled "I Am From," by George Ella Lyon. She then asked us to take a few minutes and to write our version of this same poem. It was easy for me to write at this time. Mrs. Stromberg encouraged us to write about life as it was now for us, to write about our innermost feelings. She brought back memories of these kinds of instructions from my first college English teacher, who really taught me to write. It was nice to remember back to this much loved teacher who helped me to learn to communicate on paper. I was happy to discover that writing poetry could come back to me.

I wrote the following in just a half-hour sitting in that class with other Cancer people:

I'm From . . .

By Beverly Stacy Dittmer
September 4, 2003

I'm from strong Texas stock—
From a farm lady (my grandmother) who raised six children by herself,
From a dirt share cropper who benefited from the death of a son in World War II by
    receiving enough money to finally buy land,
From a man (my father) who worked carrying a gun in a Texas oil boom town.
People who made their way with little help.

I'm from the land—
Hard, bare, white, hot West Texas desert,
Where the sandstorms blew so thick that the sun couldn't shine
    And it was dark at noon,
Where the sand hung in the air and piled up everywhere inside and out.
There was no escape from it.

I'm from schools of learning—
Where a universe of books, writing, mathematics, and science opened the world for
    me,
Where I learned to stand alone without my parents,
So that I could see beyond the dirt and the land and my heritage.
I could fly!

I'm from being a mother—
Times when I cried with my children because it was so hard,
Happy, laughing times with them full of singing,
Times of tiredness when my bones would be so weary that I thought that I couldn't
    do one thing more—
But I could.

Now I'm from a land of danger and monsters—
Where I walk in the darkest night of all time,
Where plans are tenuous and pain colors daily life,
Where I live with IVs, bandages, blood, and strange smelling fluids
Cancer invaded my body.

But I'm a thriver, I'm a survivor.

I'm *not* from Cancer.

    Our second exercise in this journaling session was to take something from our "I Am From . . ." poem that wasn't necessarily a person and personify it by having it write me a letter. Of course, I personified my Cancer. The following writing resulted from these instructions in this short class:

Cancer Personified

By Beverly Stacy Dittmer

September 4, 2003

Dear Beverly,

Remember when I lay hidden and undetected in your body. Your life was happy and carefree and full of activity. You were physically strong and healthy and suffered pain only when you cut your finger or burned your hand or overworked a muscle. You only took aspirin to help your heart. You took friends and family and life pretty much for granted. You told everyone that you were going to live to be a hundred and four.

Then many years ago, I got inside your body. You'll never know where I came from or why I chose you. I settled in your nice, big, soft, and fat-filled right breast. It was warm and nurturing, just like it had been when your babies suckled. In fact, I decided to make my first home just under your nipple. I settled in and slowly, quietly grew and multiplied. I didn't cause any problems. I gave you no pain. I caused no external skin distortions. I didn't change my x-ray profile from year to year. By being under your nipple, I safely hid in physical breast exams.

I concentrated on growing and hiding. As I got stronger, I decided it was time to expand. I sent out new settlers through the lymph system under your arm. I am getting ready to take over your body. Sometime soon, someone will find me, but I am strong now. I will hang on and battle. I would like to make your whole body my home. I will drink your blood, your energy, and your strength. Eventually I will kill you if I have my way.

But you found me on June 11, 2003. The war is on. I will not surrender.

Beverly's Infiltrating Lobular Carcinoma

In the third exercise in this two-hour class I titled my writing, which is part poetry and part prose, "Dark Times." It describes in a small way the depression that I felt upon finding out that I had Cancer.

Dark Times

I walk in the darkest time of my life.

I have experienced failure in not meeting my own standards—I didn't make all A's.

I have experienced the pains of nearly losing two of my babies and the birth of three.

I have experienced the fear of a dark night after midnight when I was lost in a rainstorm and alone.

I have traveled the world and have been a stranger alone in a strange land.

I have lived through the ending of a twenty-two-year marriage with a husband who did not want a divorce.

I have buried my father and my brother.

I watched my mother-in-law die of breast Cancer.

None of these "bad times" compared to the night when I lay in bed, doing my monthly breast self-exam and found the lump. My time got even darker when a month later, the surgeon told me that I had infiltrating lobular carcinoma, breast Cancer. I was in a state of shock.

How could this possibly be? I had none of the Cancer markers. No one else in my family had Cancer. I had nursed each of my children. I started my menses at twelve, the normal age. I had gone into menopause at fifty, which was also perfectly normal. How could this happen to me?

I have the perfect life—seven wonderful, productive, and fairly happy children, a good husband, and fourteen fabulous grandchildren. My husband and I are retired and live very comfortably in a home in Texas and in Colorado. I don't have time for this devastating disease. How could this be happening to me?

How will I ever learn to handle Cancer? Will I survive or will I die? If I do live, will I have a productive and a quality life? Will I die helpless and painfully? I thought other people would die, not me. How can I cope? Will I be able to stand the pain? What am I going to look like without any hair on my body? What about all the needles? Will the sun ever shine again? Please, God, let this *not* be happening to me.

Sitting in that special class that afternoon while quickly writing down my inner feelings helped me. It seemed to give me something productive from the feelings that had been nothing but bad for me before when they were hidden but very present in my mind. Writing these feelings, letting them out, somehow made them less dark and less threatening. I greatly encourage anyone who has to battle Cancer to *communicate your inner fears and feelings.* Writing about them truly makes them a little less scary.

Breakout Session "Taming Your Inner Dragons"

That same afternoon Paul attended "Taming Your Inner Dragons" and received a ten-minute relaxation massage, which of course, he really enjoyed. I don't know how he was taught to "tame his inner dragons," but he never let any of his hidden dragons of our fight against Cancer show to me. He was always a rock of strength for me.

Friday Morning Speakers

John Mendelsohn

Early Friday morning, we returned to the hotel and the conference. Our first speaker was John Mendelsohn, MD, the president of MD Anderson. He graduated from Harvard Medical School, was a graduate assistant to the man who discovered the double helix of genetic material, and later invented Arissa, a Cancer-fighting drug that used early genetics discoveries and that had only recently been made available to fight Cancers. He was an interesting, accomplished, caring, and a very competent man. Care and efficiency emanated from his being—the same caring and efficiency that I easily saw reflecting from all the people at MD Anderson.

Bob Arnot

Our second speaker was Dr. Bob Arnot. At this time, we had all seen him on NBC. He was currently NBC's special foreign correspondent and reported from the front lines during the Iraq War (the first Iraq War—Desert Storm). In his work in Iraq, he went into downtown Baghdad and discovered the Central Baghdad Hospital, where nearly all of the patients had been evacuated. However, all of the Cancer patients had been left behind. This situation put Dr. Bob into the immediate action mode. He used his NBC correspondent's position with the American military and managed to get a few seats on a medical evacuation helicopter in which to take a few of these "left behind" patients to safety out of Iraq.

However, this action left him with the devastating job of choosing which Cancer patients that would be sent out. What a horrible thing to have to do! At that time, he also managed to get out a few children who had Cancer to Jordan to a new Cancer Center. Since that emergency time, he has set up a foundation to try to get more of the Iraq Cancer children out of the country. It was exciting listening to the magnificent work that he performed to help the Iraqi children. Dr. Bob was a handsome, caring, adventurous, and philanthropic man. He spoke with feeling and sincerity and won his audience over in the first few minutes of his speech. I hoped that I would get the opportunity to follow his works and life. I certainly brought home one of his books.

Ted Kennedy

The next speaker on Friday morning was Mr. Ted Kennedy, Jr. (son of the senior senator from Massachusetts), who told us all about his Cancer experience. At the age of twelve, Ted had a Cancer on his leg that required that his leg be amputated from his knee down. His doctor, Dr. Norman Jaffe, MD, in Boston, Massachusetts, where Ted was treated, later came to work at MD Anderson. Ted and Dr. Jaffe grew very close. Ted's story of having Cancer in this very famous family and its aftermath of treatments was touching. Ted was being treated during his family's public time, making being down or sick almost impossible. Mr. Kennedy grew up, however, and survived his Cancer despite the many difficulties he experienced being from such a prominent family. His Cancer has never recurred. He is a lawyer now and focuses his work with the disabled and handicapped. He said that Cancer altered his life forever (for the good).

After his talk, microphones were opened up from the floor for questions, and there were some interesting ones for Ted. He was asked if there were any Republicans in the giant Kennedy clan, and he replied, "Yes, his name is Arnold." Of course, this answer brought a lot of laughter. He was also asked if he would ever run for president. He replied that he enjoyed being with his family and his children right now. I guessed that we would all just have to wait to see if he ever runs. After hearing him talk, I was convinced that Ted, Jr., was one of the "good Kennedys."

Roundtable Discussions

For our lunch that day, we met for roundtable discussions. The dining area was set up with big round tables. Each table was labeled with a big sign. You were supposed to sit at the table that fit your description. Some of the labels read breast Cancer, lung Cancer, ovarian Cancer, caregivers, sarcoma, and prostate Cancer. I, of course, sat down at the breast Cancer table, and Paul sat at the caregivers' table. I found that it was interesting and helpful to talk with other women who had already gone through breast Cancer.

When everyone found out that I had just been diagnosed, they took me under their wing and advised and counseled me. *Cancer seems to break down the walls between strangers so that immediately you are friends.* Everyone opens up and gets close quickly at a Cancer conference. This was the first time in the unplanned journey that I had experienced a group breast Cancer session. It would not be the last time that I talked and benefited from the care and the wisdom of other breast Cancer survivors.

BREAST CANCER: THE UNPLANNED JOURNEY - LESSONS LEARNED

Breakout Session "Am I Done Yet?"

Friday afternoon, I attended the breakout session entitled "Am I Done Yet? Continued Cancer Screening and Early Detection of Other Cancers in Cancer Survivors." This session stressed the fact that *you are never completely done with Cancer. You must listen to your body* and let your doctor know of any of your suspicions. Cancer does reoccur, sometimes many years later. If you can catch it early, you can stop it. There are lots of Cancer survivors at this conference. Some are Cancer-free, and many continue the battle against Cancer, but they all seem to live.

Breakout Session "Health Profiles of Cancer Survivors"

That Friday afternoon, Paul attended "Health Profiles of Cancer Survivors." He didn't tell me much about this session but did indicate that since I was reading all of the Cancer survivor books, I probably knew these profiles. Knowing the profiles of Cancer survivors helps you emulate actions and ideas in your own life. You should *use these Cancer survivors to model your own life from.*

Breakout Session "Chemobrain: Cognitive Impairment"

Paul also attended a session entitled "Chemobrain: Cognitive Impairment." This topic was interesting to me because before this conference I didn't know that it was even a word. My spell checker on my computer at that time (2003) did not recognize *chemobrain* as a real word. However, apparently, it is a fact that chemotherapy most definitely affects your brain and your thinking. I knew that when I was so stressed and depressed early in this disease, I was not able to make good decisions. In Colorado, I laid everything off on Paul. He got us packed and got us back to Texas. I was not able to organize and pack and do things that I ordinarily would do almost automatically. I wondered what I would be like after having had several sessions of chemotherapy. I thought that I would rely even more on Paul, and I did. What a load for him!

We learned a little about chemobrain from that session. However, I learned much more about it in the spring of 2004 when I was deep into chemotherapy. My cognitive powers were almost completely destroyed. For example, I could not learn how to operate a new Apple computer. I had learned numerous new computer systems when I worked for AT&T and NCR. I was a "computer person." I had no trouble remembering new procedures and new ways before I got Cancer. No matter what notes I took in the spring of 2004, I just couldn't seem to catch on to this new system. In the fall of 2004, when the chemotherapy was over, I was able to move around in this new computer without too much difficulty. I think that the effects of chemobrain were very real, and I think that now my brain has recovered from the effects of the destructive chemicals of chemotherapy.

Breakout Session "Coping with the Fear of Reoccurrence"

My second session that Friday afternoon was entitled "Coping with the Fear of Reoccurrence." I didn't really get an answer or a plan for this fear in the class. The speaker talked about recognizing the signs of depression, fear, etc., and this was helpful. I also found out that MD Anderson has a huge support network that is available to its patients. I decided that I needed to get into this support network and to use its many aids and counselors if I was going to be able to deal with this "new" fear. I had been so tied up with dealing with the fears that accompany the diagnosis of Cancer that I hadn't really thought down the road far enough to realize that I might someday have to deal with its reoccurrence.

Friday Evening Banquet

Friday night, we enjoyed a banquet with this large Cancer survivor group. The master of ceremonies was Greg Hurst, the news anchor at channel 11 in Houston. We enjoyed a performance by a banjo band. Lastly, we were entertained for over an hour by Robert Schimmel, a humorist. He is an award-winning stand-up comedian and writer who had just been featured with his own HBO special and had finished shooting the pilot for his own network sitcom *Schimmel* when in 2000, he was diagnosed with non-Hodgkin's lymphoma, a Cancer of the immune system. He went to the Mayo Clinic in Phoenix and received treatment. Of course, he had to forfeit his network sitcom. He told us about his fight to gain his life and his health back. He kept us laughing and laughing and laughing. Someone who did not have Cancer might have thought that some of the jokes were black humor. But to someone with Cancer, his jokes were just real life and were very funny.

Fortunately, Paul and I stayed Friday night at the hotel. We went up to our room after the banquet and enjoyed watching the ladies tennis final match of the US Open before we went to sleep. I don't think that I have seen a finer ladies tennis match. So even though we were up until after midnight, we were very entertained and happy. Those rich, fun-filled moments were precious at this time in my life.

Talk by a Comedian Entitled "Don't Look Back—We're Not Going that Way"

Saturday was another busy day at the conference. The session opened with a talk entitled "Don't Look Back—We're Not Going that Way" by the comedian Marcia Wallace. It was the story of her life and about her husband's death from Cancer. She told of her pain, her struggles, and her hardships being married to a man who was dying from Cancer. She explained that if she was ever going to be happy again, she had to pick up her things and just go on. In her comedic style, she entertained us and led us to realize that *life goes on, always.*

Survival Panel Discussion

We then listened to a survivor panel discussion. Two of the panelists were doctors at MD Anderson and told very personal human tales of their successful battles with Cancer and how Cancer had changed their lives. The only lady on the panel, Mary Sharkey, was a two-year survivor of pancreatic Cancer. It was amazing that she had been "cured" of this death-sentencing Cancer. It was caught early, and she was now vibrant and healthy and strong. She was young and was raising her lively family.

The doctors' stories were impressive and encouraging. I always thought that doctors never got anything like Cancer, but this discussion showed me that my thoughts were entirely incorrect. They were just as susceptible to this horrible disease as we were, and they suffered from it just as we did. The lady's story (Mary Sharkey), however, made me feel very encouraged. What a hope for me! If MD Anderson doctors and God could cure pancreatic Cancer that was almost always a sentence of death, surely they would be able to cure my stage 2 breast Cancer.

Breakout Session "Breakthroughs in the Treatment of Breast Cancer"

On Saturday afternoon, we had more breakout sessions. I attended one entitled "Breakthroughs in the Treatment of Breast Cancer." It was very enlightening. I was absolutely amazed to find out what they have discovered and how they treat breast Cancer today. My only prior experience with breast Cancer had come in 1983, when my mother-in-law, who had been fighting her Cancer for about four years, succumbed in a painful death. If she had been fighting her Cancer today, I think that she might have lived longer with less pain and disabilities. It was encouraging to see the many new treatments that have been developed.

It was also interesting hearing the comments and the questions from the women in the room. I was sitting by a lady who had infiltrating carcinoma in situ (a precancerous condition that doctors today do not even remove). She had the in situ removed from her breast and was very concerned about its reoccurrence. There were other women in the room who had stage 4 breast Cancer. They asked questions about their continuing treatment, and I was gratified to know that they were living normal lives even with their Cancers.

I discovered that there was much to learn in the field of breast Cancer, and I resolved to set about to acquire more knowledge. *Knowledge,* I felt, *helped to dispel those monsters that crept up in hard times.*

Survivors' Birthday Party

An eventful ending to this most informative seminar occurred on Saturday afternoon, when we all enjoyed a survival birthday party. The party began by recognizing Cancer survivors. The master of ceremonies asked everyone who had survived Cancer for one to three years to stand, and then he had the survivors of three to five years stand. He went on to recognize survivors of five to ten years and then ten to twenty years, and finally, he asked those who had survived Cancer for over twenty years to stand. There were only about ten people who stood for the over twenty years, but there was one forty-year survivor of Cancer. I was again amazed at the numbers of these seemingly normal Cancer survivors.

The master of ceremonies then asked for anyone who had just been recently diagnosed to stand. There was one other person besides me who stood. There were only two of us "newbies" in this large crowd. Where were all the other newly diagnosed Cancer patients? I supposed that they were all busy fighting this disease. Because I had been given a sabbatical (a time of resting and healing before I had my double mastectomy), I had time to find out about and to attend this wonderful conference.

This time had been very beneficial to me in my journey. I will always thank MD Anderson for putting it on and for making it available to me just at this crucial time in my life. This conference is put on each year in the fall, and they celebrated its fifteenth anniversary that year (2003). Apparently, Cancer survivors come back to attend year after year. It surely was nice to know that there are so many survivors of Cancer who lead normal, active, and seemingly healthy lives.

My Learnings from This Seminar

When the seminar ended at five that Saturday afternoon, we each got a small piece of a huge birthday cake. We had discovered that most of the 630 people at this conference had endured Cancer at some time in their lives, and some are still enduring Cancer. *In the general population, one out of every three people will have Cancer today. One of every eight women will have breast Cancer. Cancer is a fact of life today.* During this conference, I accepted the fact that I am the *one* in those eight women who has Cancer—and that I can survive Cancer. I now think that *Cancer is a chronic disease rather than a terminal disease.* How's that for "coming around"?

I felt more hopeful that Saturday after completing the conference than I had since I found out that I had Cancer. I knew for sure by the examples of these many unimportant and important people that *life goes on, and I would go on with it* (even if I had to fight Cancer on the journey).

It had been a very busy and informative time. I had seen lots of people who had, it seemed, learned how to live their lives fully with Cancer. The knowledge and the experiences that I gained at this seminar made my adventure through this disease easier and less fearful.

I would use these Cancer survivors as models. I would follow their lead in learning how to live my life fully with Cancer, I hoped. The death monster still lived in the depths of my soul, but after being in this seminar for a few days, it lay quiet and still.

Chapter 19

COMPLETING ALL MY "BEFORE SURGERY" TASKS—WAITING WITH THE MONSTER

My Physical Condition at This Time

Again, from my newsletter, I reported on my physical condition as follows:

> I am still on my sabbatical. I started to feel halfway decent again about August 30. I got stronger each day until now I am nearly back to my old normal self. I still have a breast that is open, that still bleeds, and that drains a little. Paul is poking in about ten inches of gauze/tape each evening. The actual poking doesn't hurt now. Either I have gotten used to it or my breast has healed enough that it isn't so sore. It just continually reminds me that it is an open aggravation. I feel good. I don't think that the surgeon will postpone my mastectomy any longer. I think that he will feel pleased with the way my hematoma has healed.

Seeing My Mother Again

I set about after the Houston MD Anderson seminar to see all of my family and friends as soon as I got to feeling better. My ninety-one-year-old mother was first on my list of people to visit. She lives in Coleman, Texas, and doesn't travel much. I talked to her every week by phone, but I hadn't seen her since we had left Texas in the spring. Since Paul was very busy completing chores and work at our house, he felt that he could not take the time to drive with me to Coleman. I did not feel like I could go by myself, so I asked my friend, Mary Lee Hamisch, if she could accompany me. She graciously accepted and even wanted to drive her car. So Mary Lee and I left on Tuesday, August 26, to drive to Coleman.

It was a wonderful to spend time with Mother and my sister, Karen. My sister had already gone through chemotherapy treatments in 1998, when she battled lupus. She told me all about how her treatments were. I could ask any questions that I wanted, and it was enlightening. I hoped that my treatments weren't going to be as harsh as hers had been. However, if she could do them, surely I could do them also. She told stories similar to the ones that I had read in Lance Armstrong's book. She also told me that every day that she received her actual chemo treatments in the chemotherapy treatment room, she thanked God that she only had lupus.

Lance Armstrong also got through his Cancer and was grateful for having experienced it. Amy Givler, another of the Cancer survivor writers, also stated that although she wouldn't wish Cancer on anyone, she was thankful for the changes that occurred in her because of the battle with her Cancer.

I don't feel thankful that I have breast Cancer. I guess that I am just not far enough down my road yet to appreciate the experience. I am not yet ready to thank God for this breast Cancer. Maybe I will someday.

My mother was stressed because of her worry for me. She was a kind, loving mother and would do anything to help me. I truly wish that she had been healthy and strong so that she could have come to care for me. No one ever took care of me like my mother did. If I had to be sick, the best way to do it was under her care. She always knew just what to do to soothe the pain or the ache. I knew that I had to do this disease without her physical care, but I knew that she was sending me her love and her care from long distance.

That evening, my sister stuffed the clean gauze into my wound following my voice directions. It was a really good time of being together.

Seeing Lilli

On Monday, September 1, I kept Lilli (age six), one of my favorite grandchildren, a whole day while her daddy, Paul Damian number six son, worked. We had a grand time, and I spent the afternoon making her a treasured pig pillow. I allowed her to choose the fabric from my storage boxes. I showed her how we cut out the pattern and then the material, and finally, I sewed up the pig while she put together puzzles on the floor by my sewing machine. It was kind of a long project, but she seemed totally pleased with the product that she took home with her that evening.

After lunch that day, I insisted that I would be sick if I did not get my nap, so Lilli sat on the bed with me for an hour. She watched cartoons and played with a special toy, my Mouse House, while I rested and dozed. What a wonderful grandchild she is, and what a wonderful afternoon I shared with her!

Going Back to Colorado

We made a short visit back to Colorado on September 7. I wrote about the plans for that trip by saying the following:

> We miss Colorado so much that we have squeezed in a trip back. I want everyone in Durango to remember me happy and strong, not weak and sad like I was when I left. I want us to enjoy a "Boobs Begone" potluck lunch. I want to hug and to greet all of my mountain friends. I want to see my magnificent and cragged La Plata Mountains one more time. I want to walk in the cool air and enjoy the brisk fall mornings. If the Aspen are turning anywhere, I want to drive out to see them. I want to sit a moment in "my seat" at Christ the King Lutheran Church. (We probably can't be there for the Sunday service, but I want to visit anyway. God is there all of the time so it will be okay.)

Paul and I had spent Saturday night, September 6, with Jeff and Liz and Erica in Houston. Sunday morning, we got up at four and went to the airport. We caught a flight at 6:45 a.m. to Denver and then on to Durango. It was so nice to see the rugged Rockies as we got close to Durango. The sky was full of clouds, and we couldn't see the mountains earlier when we came into Denver. From there, the winds and United Airlines carried us swiftly across the mountains to our Colorado home, Durango. We made it to Colorado just as I had planned. One of our Durango friends arrived to pick us up as soon as we landed. She dropped me at our church on the way through town as she drove Paul out to our house to pick up our car. He immediately got into our car and drove back into town so that he even caught the last of our Sunday service. What a joy it was for me to be in this wonderful spiritual home church and to see my church friends and family here in Colorado one last time before I went back to Houston to begin the second half of my unplanned journey!

After the Sunday morning service, we bought a few groceries and settled into our house. The yard was green and lush (for Colorado). The La Plata Mountains, the Ponderosas, and all the things that we could see outside of our windows were beautiful. Because Durango had not yet had a freeze, our tomato vines were full of green tomatoes. Our geraniums were gorgeous. The natural world was rich and full at this season of harvest. This world was ready and prepared for the cold winter that lay just ahead. I hoped that I was ready for the next phase of my Cancer battle, the next leg of the unplanned journey.

I, of course, got on the phone when we arrived home and called friends. We enjoyed dinner that evening with our friends, Raul and Noeli Galvan. It was cold that night, and it felt secure and comforting to snuggle beneath our down comforter in our Colorado bed.

Bev's Boobs' Begone Bash

We awoke early on Monday morning to find our gorgeous Colorado day gray and cloudy. It was drizzling rain. However, I couldn't let a little rain ruin my last full day in Colorado, so we jumped up and went into town to enjoy a water aerobics class with our friends, the Mermaids. After a time of exercise and visiting, we went over to my friend's house, Therese Teiber, to enjoy Bev's Boobs' Begone potluck. My good friends, Therese and Marge Rebovich, had done a lot of work preparing for this big event. They had only a very short time to plan everything because I hadn't decided that I could come back to Durango until just a few days earlier. They asked everyone to bring food that was related to and shaped like boobs. This event was planned to be a happy, light-hearted tribute to me and my boobs, as they knew that I was going through a life-altering change very soon and would no longer have my boobs.

By lunchtime, the morning drizzle of rain had turned into a full-fledged rain storm and the sky was pouring down rain, but Therese was prepared. She had moved her banquet tables from her lovely lawn to under her carport on her front porch. She had made a place for all of the food on her kitchen counters inside. We all had room to sit outside under the carport while the musical rain serenaded our party with its wonderful lyrical sounds. There were no gray spirits among the attendees at this assemblage. Nearly all of my Colorado water aerobic (the Mermaids) friends came to the party. We had quite a crowd.

Therese had decorated her house and had a 1959 vintage very flat-chested baby doll sitting on her table, with a two-piece pink bikini on. The doll was showing off that it was okay to be flat-chested. Therese got white Styrofoam egg cartons and cut them across by twos. She used brown markers to mark the center on the outside of the egg holders so that each set of two looked like a set of boobs. These Styrofoam boobs were the party favors, and each attendee took a set home with them.

Therese prepared to serve a delicious spaghetti squash that she had grown in her garden. In order to follow the theme of the party, she cut the squash in half, baked the two half shells, and then scraped out the insides to season and to serve. She took the shells that were left and turned them over and decorated the outside shells with two cherries that were also cut in half and stuck onto the squash shells with toothpicks. The two inverted and decorated squash shells looked very much like two breasts.

Another friend brought two mounds of potato salad that were also decorated with cherries in the top center so that her dish of potato salad looked like boobs. We all had a big chuckle over the boob-related foods. The food was great as it always is. Everyone toasted to my health and well-being. After filling our plates inside, we sat down at the tables outside in the fifty-degree weather, with the rain pouring down all around us. Our bodies may have been a little chilled but our hearts were filled with great warmth and love.

Marge and Darlene Bliss had made and decorated a huge cake that was made in the shape of a curvy lady's body with a strapless purple swimsuit on. There were two large mounds of cake decorated to perfection in tan icing to resemble two luscious breasts. It was a most interesting and appropriate cake. We were celebrating my boobs and consequently the loss of my boobs. When this cake appeared at the end of our meal, we all laughed and laughed.

After we had all eaten our fill of the delicious food and cake, the girls got up and sang a song they had written for me. It was entitled "I Got Along Without You Before I Had You, I'll Get Along Without You Now." The lyrics to the song were from the old song, "I got along without you before I met you, and I'll get along without you now." The *you* that this special song referred to was my boobs. The girls had taken the old song and rewritten the words just to cover my mastectomy. Their words to the song were:

> You got along without them before you had them,
> You can get along without them now!
>
> You got along without them before you had them,
> You can get along without them now!
>
> They have served you well!
> You have *worn* them well!
>
> But
>
> You got along without them before you had them
> You can get along without them now!
>
> They have just plain gone to he—!
> So it's so long, farewell.
>
> Our Beverly won't be undone
>
> So it's "So long, Boobs, be gone!"
>
> She got along without you before she had you
> And she'll get along without you now!

The lyrics were encouraging and hilarious. I laughed until I cried. We all giggled and hugged and openly expressed our love for one another. I managed to talk through my tears and to tell everyone that I knew my journey ahead would be much better knowing that I had such caring and supportive friends. It was a magnificent party, and even though the cold rain fell all around us just a few feet away, it did nothing to daunt our happy spirits.

My good friend, Therese, wrote about the party and said, "The event was such a great success. It provided us all a chance to tell Beverly how much we loved and supported her. It gave her the opportunity to say farewell to us before embarking on this unplanned journey. We all cried and hugged. It was a great day, one that none of us will ever forget. There will be a great life after Cancer."

I really enjoyed this party and my final farewell to my Colorado friends. I had just laughed and laughed and laughed. This is the way that I had wanted to leave my friends. I wanted them to remember me laughing and happy. The party was a great achievement because it helped me to appear to be strong, and it allowed me to see all of my friends in a very short period of time. Durango got a record-breaking amount of rain that afternoon (3.1 inches), but the rain was nothing compared to the problems that I would soon be facing.

After the party, Paul drove me up the mountains toward Silverton, and I got to see the golden Aspen before winter set in. It had been a happy and successful trip. The next morning, we closed our house down a second time that year and left for the airport to fly back to Grapevine. I was satisfied that if I died, the last memory my friends would have of me was a happy one.

Talking to John

On Thursday, September 11, I spoke on the phone with number five son, John. We talked for quite a while, and I was able on the phone to discuss my disease with him rationally (without me crying). He told me that he didn't like to deal with something like Cancer for his mom but that he was all right with it. He said that I shouldn't worry about him and that he would try to be better in the future about calling me and talking to me about the Cancer. I do think that he was all right after our talk. He was one of the people that I had on my list to be sure and talk to before my surgery. He was a pilot for United Airlines and had to fly that weekend, so he had to miss our big family gathering.

After I had completed my Cancer battle, John decided that he wanted to train to become a physician's assistant so that he could help people. I don't know whether my having Cancer influenced him or not, but I do know that I was very concerned about John's acceptance of the disease in my life.

Unexpected, Unplanned Illness

Friday evening, September 12, before we left for Houston, I became very ill. I vomited and had diarrhea all at the same time. I felt like I had fever. I didn't want to get sick and not be able to complete all of my visiting plans. I didn't want to get sick and not be able to have my mastectomy surgery on Monday. I think that my hidden fears had just bubbled over to upset my body. My nerves had taken control of my body against my mind's wishes. I went to bed Friday night fearing the worst things, but God must have healed my body during the night. I woke up Saturday morning feeling much better.

The Last Day in Grapevine, Saturday, September 13

Saturday dawned bright and sunny and hot. I had to prepare my Texas sheet cake (a very moist and delicious chocolate cake) for Mary Joy's birthday cake, and I also had to make her very favorite dessert, banana pudding. I ran through the house, doing some cleaning in preparation for our leaving early Sunday morning for Houston, knowing I wouldn't be back for a while. We arranged for our neighbors to put out feed for Mr. Boots while we were gone. I dressed for my last day at home.

I had arranged with our family photographer to have a picture-taking session. We met him right after lunch, and he took numerous shots of Paul and me. I had simply told Paul that I wanted to take a professional family photograph. Inside, my thoughts were that I was taking this photograph so that the kids could remember me as I wanted them to remember me—healthy (at least I looked that way on the outside now), with my boobs and my hair, and when I was happy. Since I thought deep down inside that I would never be this way again and that I really might die, it was very important to get the photograph taken.

Our old family photographer met us at a lovely little Grapevine park, and we had pictures made with azaleas blooming in the background. There was something wrong with our Texas flowers at that moment. They had their seasons all confused. The gardenias in my yard were blooming again just like they did in the spring. These two spring flowers were blooming on September 13. I should have taken this as a special blessing from God. I was getting to enjoy beautiful spring blossoming flowers in the fall. I was too busy getting things done that day to stop and to smell the gardenias and the azaleas. Shame on me! I hadn't learned that "stop and smell the roses" lesson yet.

Our picture did turn out really pretty, however, with the blooming pink azaleas in the background almost a perfect match to the pink dress that I had chosen to wear. I have proof of the mixed-up flowers and God's hidden blessing to me in this picture. And we did get this task accomplished even though our day was very busy.

This was an election day, and feeling like I do about voting, I told Paul that we had to go to the polls to vote. This happened to be the weekend of the Grapevine Grapefest, and our little town was absolutely full of people. In trying to find the voting place, we got all tied up in traffic. This was not the way that I had planned to spend the last of my valuable free time, so I got out of our car and directed traffic so that we could escape the car snarl up. People looked at me a little funny, but traffic was just all balled up and no one was going anywhere quickly. With some direction, all of the cars started moving. Paul was a little embarrassed by my aggressiveness, but I was not going to miss something that I had planned to complete today when I had so little time left because of a traffic jam.

BREAST CANCER: THE UNPLANNED JOURNEY - LESSONS LEARNED

When we finally found our voting place despite all of the traffic in town and having the wrong voting site information, most of the afternoon had been all used up. Nothing so far in this disease had been easy, so I wasn't really discouraged about these last two chores of mine being difficult. A lot of things that should be laws are voted on as constitutional amendments in Texas. In this way, at times, the voters get to actually pass laws.

This Saturday, we had before the electorate Proposition 12, which proposed to limit the noneconomic costs that patients could sue for in malpractice suits. I very much wanted this proposition to pass, even though our major papers came out against this issue. I felt like the turnout for this election would be low (there were only constitutional amendments on the ballot), and therefore, my vote would be valuable. We had two doctors in the family, Mary Joy and her husband, Tarl, and we wanted them to move back to Texas when they finished their residencies in Detroit, Michigan. It was important that Texas pass this legislation to help protect doctors from huge medical malfeasance suits. I wanted Mary Joy to move closer to our homes. Paul and I finally made it to the right poll and cast our votes.

We then set off to drive over to Mansfield (forty-five minutes away) so that we could go to Mary Joy's birthday party. We arrived at the party at 5:20 p.m.—the last ones to get there. Mary Lee Hamisch and her husband, Frank, had decorated their house in a Texas motif. He had barbequed a brisket, and we brought a cooked ham. There were lots of other good food and drinks. I owe Mary Lee another huge debt of gratitude for her hosting this party at her house. It was much easier for me this way. I got to spend time with most of my children and grandchildren. Time had been so short in this one-month sabbatical, which I had enjoyed, that I wanted to make the very best use of every moment.

In attendance that early evening were James and Cristi Hyde, number four son and his family, Jamie, Alli, Ben, and Garrett; Shelley Hyde, wife of number five son, John, and his family, Madeline, and Gabby; Paul Hyde, number six son, and his wife Stephanie; and Mary Joy, number seven child. My ex-husband, Jimmy Hyde, and his wife, Linda, were even there. I was so happy to have James there because he works all over the country, and I hadn't gotten to see him often. I was able to sit down with him and to have a nice talk. We both agreed to put the problem that we had two years ago behind us. We talked about his radiation treatments when he had Hodgkin's disease. He is the tallest of my three boys at six feet three. We took photographs of James, Paul, and me. I was surrounded by two giants because I am only five feet seven and they are both several inches over six feet tall.

We were entertained by the antics of the little ones, and Grandmother B (me) had a fabulous time. Mary Joy had birthday cake and ice cream and banana pudding. Ben, one of my grandchildren, and I played "tea" together and drank water that he got to pour into little neat liquor glasses that he was very careful not to break. I taught him to hold up his fifth finger when he drank daintily. We drank the plain water, but we pretended that it was delicious tea, and it was fun. The party was simple, and the food was very good. But the most important thing was for me to be with my children and my grandkids one last time.

We took lots of pictures. It was warm, the evening sun was shining brightly, and I enjoyed a very good time. Far too soon, it was time to leave. I said good-bye to everyone. I hugged them all and received many kisses from the grandkids. They didn't really know what was going on, but they knew that Grandmother B was very sick. Mary Joy went home with us to Grapevine, and I stayed one last night in my Texas home.

Mary Joy attempted to encourage me that evening by telling me something new about Cancer:

> After attending the MD Anderson seminar on Cancer, I had told Mary Joy that I had decided that Cancer was a chronic disease, not a terminal one. Well, my doctor daughter corrected me this evening. She assured me that *Cancer was a curable disease* and that she was looking for a cure for me.

Hooray for my supporter! She was sure that I would beat this stuff! Cancer was a reality in my life, and standing in her comforting and loving presence that evening, I was determined to beat and survive it.

Sunday September 14, 2003, the Last Day of My Sabbatical

The next morning, we got up, loaded the car, and headed out down I-45 to Houston. I lay in the back and napped on the way down, saving my strength to enjoy the hours that lay ahead before the surgery. It was nice to rest. Mary Joy and Paul visited in the front seat while I dozed, and the time dozing, resting, and listening to their conversation was good.

We arrived in Spring, at Jeff and Liz's house, just about lunchtime. My high school girlfriend, Sharon Reynolds Kimbrel, and her husband arrived a few minutes after us. It was granddaughter Erica's twelfth birthday lunch, and her mother, Liz, outdid herself by having prepared green enchilada's, frijoles rancheros, and mud pie. We all sat down and enjoyed a delicious meal. It was so nice to be with Sharon again. We talked and talked in an effort to catch up on all of the news.

After lunch, Paul, MJ, Sharon, Jeff, Liz, Erica, and I got into our cars and drove to Friendswood, which is a suburb that is in the Southeast part of Houston. We arrived at Peter Dittmer's house, number two son. His wife, Sondra, had prepared a big baked ham that she served in a kind of formal sit-down dinner. They had recently purchased a big new house, and everyone enjoyed seeing it and visiting a while. I had enjoyed a busy, full, food-filled day topped over with celebrations—Erica's birthday, Sharon's birthday, and Sondra and Peter's anniversary. It was nice to see nearly all of the Dittmer clan again before my surgery. I had now completed my "To Do Before Surgery" list!

BREAST CANCER: THE UNPLANNED JOURNEY - LESSONS LEARNED

After the dishes were all cleaned, we all settled in. I spent a restful evening surrounded loving family and friends. It was a rainy night with lightning and thunder raging outside when I took a luxurious soaking bath in Sondra's big jet tub. I think that God was helping me to prepare. It was violent and scary outside with the storms and the pouring rain, and I was safely surrounded by my loving family in a protected place where I could prepare for the next day of surgery. I was wrapped in the strength and comfort of my support team. I had used my sabbatical, my "feel good" time, to do the important things—to visit my family and my friends. I wanted to try to see everyone one more time before I started the serious part of my battle. I think a good lesson that I would like to share might go something like this:

> *Take advantage of any sabbatical time that you have. See your friends and family. Rest your mind and body so that your spirit can be strengthened. Use every moment, and don't waste any of the "good" time. The battle lies ahead and may be difficult.*

I had certainly tried to follow this lesson. I had visited my mother, my sister, and my niece in Coleman. I saw my niece's new twin babies. I visited with my Colorado friends again for a happy parting and a celebration with a "Boobs Begone" party. I had visited with nearly all of my children and grandchildren one last time.

I went to bed that last night, hoping that I had left everyone with a picture of a happy, controlled, strong lady. I hoped that I was girded with my shield and sword and was ready to fight, beginning with the upcoming mastectomy. I still ignored that unmentioned horrible monster of fear that lay in my belly, growling.

Chapter 20

GATHER YOUR SUPPORT TEAM

My Support Staff

Early on in the unplanned journey, people (friends, family, and friends of friends) gathered around me. I was amazed at how quickly people found out about my Cancer and then got on the bandwagon behind me. I don't believe there was a single day that passed in which I didn't receive at least one "get well" card or several "get well" e-mails. I received flowers, small gifts, and other reminders that my support team was always there.

When I was doing all of the Cancer book reading, several threads of similarity ran through them. One of these threads was that having multiple social contacts and supports improved one's survival odds. Without a great deal of effort on my part—except maybe by setting up a regular communication system—my support system was established. I set up the communications system by establishing a mailing list on my computer in early August, just after I discovered that my Cancer battle was going to be long and complicated. I could easily send out an e-mail asking for special prayers, which I often did. There are Web sites today that support daily blogs for people who are fighting illnesses. There are easy and effective ways to construct a format for your support staff. Take advantage of all the tools that are available. My lesson would be *gather your support team and use them often.*

Thanks to My Companion

Of course, one of my biggest supporters was my husband, Paul Dittmer. How does one thank someone like him? During this year of my life when I battled Cancer, he was patient, present, and always caring. He walked the road right beside me. He was my continuous friend and companion and was a very special caregiver. I was blessed, and I learned how to walk this unplanned journey one little step at a time with Paul behind me, pushing me on, or beside me, holding my hand, or in front of me, hollering at me to "Hurry up and come on." He had dedicated his life at this time to helping me beat Cancer.

Thanks to My Doctor Daughter

The second member of my medical committee was my very busy daughter, Mary Joy, and she was a big member of my support team also. I had gotten to enjoy spending a little bit of time with Mary Joy on Wednesday, September 10, just before my mastectomy surgery, when she and Tarl spent the night with us. We enjoyed some of our fabulous "girl talks," and it became very clear to me that it hurt her deeply to think about me hurting. She sensed my fear and was therefore afraid for me. She loved me and showed that love at every turn. It was truly a joy and a real help to have her around. In my recovery after the surgery, she was my own private doctor who stayed with me through that long first night and cared for me with the love that only a daughter or a mother can give. She took time out from her busy life as a resident in medical school to come and to help me. I am very thankful!

I was ready. The surgery was scheduled for me to enter at 5:00 a.m., Monday, September 15. After this surgery, we would know exactly where the Cancer was, and the doctors would know how to treat it. The Cancer battle was finally about to enter a very big and new stage.

Chapter 21

PRIVATE FEELINGS

My Very Private Thoughts

I had feared this surgery from the depth of my soul. Despite everything that I could do, it was finally time to meet this monster Cancer head on. On Friday and Saturday mornings, before traveling back to Houston, I had clung to Paul for a few minutes when we were lying together in bed in the early morning and cried. I cried because I didn't want to have this surgery. I cried because I knew that my life was going to change in big ways after this surgery. I cried because from the bottom of my heart, I was afraid. But I said no words to him about this, and he didn't ask.

Mary Joy confided after my surgery that she sensed that I thought that I was going to die during this surgery. This surgery seemed different and much harder than any of the other earlier surgeries that I had undergone. The hysterectomy and bladder tack (2000), and the rectum repair (2001), I had initiated and planned. After I began the unplanned journey, the first and second lumpectomies were done in an effort to rid my body of the Cancer. I always thought that each one of them was going to achieve that goal. The hematoma clean-out surgery was done to stop pain and infection. Now I was having the *big* surgery, the double mastectomy, in a final effort to get rid of the Cancer.

My body was now tired and battered. I had been in the Cancer fight for a while and had not scored well. The mastectomies were necessary, I knew, but I surely did not want to have them. My scurry of activity of visiting and doing things was a cover up to hide my fear. The active time was over now, and in this quiet time of the night before the surgery, I had to accept that the surgery would happen in a few hours. It was a difficult and especially scary time for me. However, I saw no way out so I walked on.

I thought and thought during my wakeful moments in the night about what my life had been. I wondered if the fears that I felt (the fears of death, disability, and pain) and had never said one single word about to anyone would come true. I wondered if this was the end of life as

I presently knew it. I lay in bed most of the tempestuous dark night and fought with the Cancer monster. About 3:00 a.m., I decided that I could now get up. I sat down and wrote a quick note to my husband, Paul.

A Note to Paul

Peter's House in Houston on Monday, September 15, 2003, 3:15 a.m.

I feel the strong need to write a tribute and a "thank you" to Paul!

Dearest Paul,

For the last seventeen years, you have been my friend and my lover.
We joined together in difficult times because we both had other partners,
But we persisted and clung together against all adversities.
We got married and put two families together and set out to live "happily ever after."
And we did—almost!

We joined our families and guided our grown and nearly grown children to friendships.
We worked and moved our separate careers so that our finances improved.
We sought and found new friends. We culled through old friendships to salvage what we could.
We traveled, and you showed me a grand, raw, and magnificent land—the West.
And we grew closer—and made memories!

Too soon we started to grow older. Your knee failed.
We both thickened. Your hair thinned and mine became streaked with gray.
Our kids went off to college, married, and began their own stories and lives.
We grew tired of working. You brought your business home and soon retired.
Our life was good—we had enough!

New wives and a new husband and grandchildren came. Our family numbers exploded.
Children and babies were everywhere. Joy and laughter and play and new life were everywhere.
We had more grandchildren than we could see on each of their birthdays.
Our sons and daughters turned into accomplished people—doctors, teachers, artists, pilots, and business owners.

Our life was full—we were proud!

And then the monster Cancer invaded my body and tenaciously garbled our lives.
The battle for survival ensued. We began "the unplanned journey."
We had to learn about our enemy. We surfed the Web, scoured scores of books, and talked to Cancer survivors.
We sought the best doctors and hospitals and came to MD Anderson in Houston.
Cancer took over—we prepared to fight!

We enlisted our core of supporters—friends, family, and friends of friends.
We gathered spiritual support and prayed and were prayed for by many people in many different churches.
I endured two lumpectomies, a clean-out surgery of a huge hematoma, with much pain and blood.
We suffered the dark times with much difficulty, deep emotional times of tears, and a time of renewing of love.
A time of *SEEING*—and the Cancer still remained!

God and the doctors gave us a two-week time of rest—a time for my body to heal and for my spirit to recuperate.
I filled that time with family visits. I saw my mother, my sister, our children, and our grandkids.
We made a family picture because my body will change from this upcoming battle.
My only daughter came from Detroit and my high school girlfriend came to support me.
We celebrated love—we are entering the fray!

Thank you for traveling with me on this life journey. You appear on every page of my book of memories during these years.
You walk beside me as I go into surgery and this long fight against Cancer. Your love and care will support me.
Your wisdom, calmness, and patience will make you a wonderful caregiver for me. No one knows me as well as you do.
Your love will shield me when the rains of chemotherapy try to drown the Cancer in my body.
We love—and I go to surgery now!

Going to the Hospital

After finishing this last note and leaving it in my things, I showered and dressed in a comfortable sweat suit so that we could leave. Mary Joy woke up by herself as I came out of the shower. Paul was up and ready on time. I don't imagine that he had slept too well himself. It was very dark as we pulled out of the driveway and headed north from Friendswood to MD

Anderson. There wasn't a moon, and you couldn't see the stars because the freeway fluorescent lights bounced their white/blue light off of the pavement and diluted any starlight that might have been present. Looking out into the black world beside the freeway reinforced my feeling of aloneness. We didn't talk much. I didn't know what to say, and I don't think that Paul or Mary Joy did either. Paul is best at doing "business/action" things. Feelings and inner thoughts are not really easy for him to share or to handle.

It wasn't crowded at MD Anderson that Monday morning at that wee early hour. We easily found a parking place and made the long walk into the hospital. We went up to the surgery entrance room, received our hospital documentation, talked to a check-in nurse, and waited to be called. We only waited about ten minutes before we were called to go back into the surgical prep room. I took off all of my clothes, put on a hospital gown, and got onto a gurney/bed. Paul was with me. Soon the anesthetist came by and put an IV needle into my hand.

Mary Joy, Sharon, and her husband, Don, came in to see me for just a minute. It was really nice to know that my family and friends were there with me. They had to have gotten up awfully early to have made it into the hospital at this hour. Dr. Ralston and his physician's assistant came by to see me. As soon as they gave me relaxing medicine, I went immediately to sleep. Whatever was going to happen was going to happen soon.

Chapter 22

Suppressing Your Fears

Waking Up with Seemingly Real Monsters

I went into surgery about 7:00 a.m. I did not get out of surgery until a little after 12:30 noon. The surgical procedures had not revealed any new obvious Cancer areas, and they had taken one sentinel lymph node under my left arm and had left the others. They had taken two residual lymph nodes from under my right arm. Everything was normal and fine. But I didn't know or feel that things were fine. I went to the recovery area after surgery and began to come out from under the anesthetic before I was told this *good* news. Later I was told that the anesthesiologist and the PA had talked to me before I came to recovery and that I had reported that I was just fine. After having talked to me for this short time, they assumed that I was okay and went on to other patients and surgeries. I have no recollection of this talk even to this day.

I started to wake up in the recovery area. I hurt everywhere. But the worst pain that I felt was in my head. I found myself in the most frightening hell-like place that I have ever experienced. It was a very real place. I had a horrible black vision of monsters and death and trouble. Amid all of this chaos in my head, I had this remembrance of the doctors talking. In my head, I saw and heard my doctor talking to another surgeon. He said, "I opened her up, and the Cancer was everywhere. I just closed her back up. She will die soon." The other doctor told him something about his patient, and then they faded away. I thought that Cancer had taken over my body. I was angry. I was irrationally scared. I hurt worse than I had ever hurt in my life. I felt like I was dying, and I knew that I had heard the doctor reinforce those feelings.

I felt that I needed to fight the Cancer battle, and I told the recovery room nurse about it. I had woken up before from surgeries with my body hurting so badly that it felt like I had been hit by a huge Mack truck. This time it felt like a fleet of Mack trucks had hit me. It hurt too badly for me to tell anyone how bad it hurt. I couldn't get up. I couldn't holler very loudly because my throat and voice just didn't work well. I thought that I knew as a fact that Cancer had taken over my body.

The recovery room nurse was working all around me. She kept telling me to calm myself down and that I had just gone through major surgery. She repeated several times that it was normal for me to feel this way. I kept telling her that this was *not* normal. She assured me that the surgery had gone fine and that they had not found any more Cancer, but nothing she said carried much weight with me. I cried and fussed. The nurse kept telling me that everything would be okay. Well, I didn't feel like I was going to be okay. My muddled drug-addled brain was playing the most awful reel of monsters and blackness that I could hardly endure. I knew that my body was filled with Cancer. I was angry and afraid all at the same time. I promised myself that I would never ever go under an anesthetic again if this was what it was going to be like. I was tossing and struggling and probably crying and calling. The nurse angrily kept telling me to settle down and wait. She repeatedly told me that everything was going to be all right. I asked for the nurse to call Dr. Ralston, my surgeon, and she said that he was in another surgery. I asked her to call Dr. Ralston's Fellow. She said that she couldn't call him either. I asked her to get Dr. Ralston's PA, but she didn't come either.

The recovery room nurse kept trying to get me to wake up. She kept asking me what my pain level was. I told her that it was fourteen. She kept saying rather angrily, "No, give me your rating on a scale from one to ten." I was very groggy, but I did finally manage to tell her that on a scale of one to ten, my pain level was fourteen. She thought that my evaluation was unimportant and went on with her work.

Mary Joy's Presence Brings Rationality

I then remembered Mary Joy. I told the nurse that my doctor daughter was in the waiting room and that I needed to see her. I told her that she must go out and get Mary Joy for me. Well, this time, she listened to my words and called for Mary Joy. Mary Joy came into the room with me. She held my hand, patted my head, and read my chart. She assured me that everything was going to be all right. After reading my chart, she told me that in just a minute, the painkillers were going to kick in and that I would start to feel better. She told me that the doctors had not found any more Cancer and that the surgery was done. How wonderful it was to have a calm, confident, loving doctor daughter at this very instant in time by my side! I needed her badly to pull me up out of that monster-filled hole that I had fallen into the moment I started to awaken from the surgery. I promised myself that I would never put myself into this kind of a situation again. I would *never* have surgery again if this were the after effects of anesthesia.

My blood pressure was 200/130. I was definitely suffering from a bad reaction wake-up. Mary Joy stayed right with me and held my hand. I knew that I would be safe with her, and I was able to slowly calm myself. The pain medication did start to work, and the horrible monsters and the bad doctor's diagnosis faded into the background. I am so thankful that Mary Joy was there to help me through this horrible "waking up" time.

Looking at this experience five years later, I think that in semiconsciousness, I had really heard some doctors talking. They obviously were not talking about me, but in my drugged state, I didn't know that. I had thought for a while that I was going to die in this surgery. This too was an irrational thought. I should have discussed these dreadful fears with someone, but I just couldn't give the fears further creditability by saying them out loud. I never talked about these fears with anyone. I did talk about them after the surgery with my counselor. We both agreed that I should have talked about these fears before I had the surgery.

My advice to my readers if you are going through Cancer is *to please talk about your innermost thoughts and fears*. When you suppress your fears and do not confront them, they may rear their ugly heads and bite you. Talking about the hidden monsters makes them easier to deal with. Bringing them out into the daylight makes them not so horribly frightening. They will not just go away by themselves. I know that I thought that if I ignored them long enough, they would go away. They didn't, however. They came out to make my wake-up from surgery *very* frightening and stressful.

Chapter 23

CONCENTRATE ON THE IMPORTANT THINGS

Settling Down to Recover

Thankfully, I lived through the recovery time. It took quite a while and lots of reassurances from Mary Joy before I could begin to feel better. Just thinking about my "wake-up experience" filled my eyes with tears, and I cringed with fear. The pain level, however, did become manageable. It had started out a fourteen on a scale of one to ten. By 4:00 p.m., I was calm and my pain level was manageable enough so that I could be moved from recovery to my room.

I was receiving morphine drips when I needed them. I couldn't move much because I had two tubes sticking out from under each arm that went into two bottles that were the size of small cantaloupes. The bottles hung below my waist from four tubes. I had a catheter above my collar bone on the left side of my chest—my central line. Paul, MJ, and Dr. Ralston had discussed this addition to my surgeries after I had gone under the anesthetic, and it was decided that to save me from having another surgery this line should be put in at this time. This central line would later be used in my chemotherapy. I also had a Foley catheter in my bladder and an IV in my hand. I didn't really have the urge to do much moving so I just lay in bed and thanked God that I was alive, that the Cancer had not spread and had not taken over my body, and that I was not in much pain. You know, at times, a person gets down *to remembering the really important things.*

I enjoyed hearing my daughter, MJ, and my old best girlfriend, Sharon, talk. I went in and out of sleep a lot during their conversations that late afternoon, and their chatter was like a soothing waterfall to my slumber. My best friend from my old high school days and my only daughter became really good friends during this time of sitting with me. Paul was there in my room also, and my shattered world was coming together again.

Paul and Sharon left about eight that night to go to Liz's house to spend the night. They were really tired since they had started the morning before 4:00 a.m.. Mary Joy thought that I should try to eat some of my liquid diet, and they brought me a tray of Jell-O. I consumed it, and found that it tasted pretty good. The orange Jell-O was absolutely delicious. I ate my liquid supper and didn't become nauseated. Mary Joy made the single chair in my room out into a bed and got sheets, a blanket, and a pillow from my nurse. Mary Joy seemed to know her way around this hospital even though she had never been in it before today. I guess when you know one hospital as a doctor, you know them all. We both settled in for the first night in the hospital after surgery. I surely felt better with Mary Joy sleeping just a couple of feet away from me.

The night flowed easily by. I took my pain medicine regularly and slept almost peacefully—it's hard to sleep too comfortably when you have to lie only on your back. Mary Joy woke up at my every move. I was amazed that she woke up every time fully cognizant and alert. She certainly wasn't that way as a teenager in our home. I guess the Doctor training and being "on call" all of the hours of the day and night had changed her sleeping habits.

My First Day After Surgery

Tuesday arrived, my first day after surgery, and I started eating a regular diet. I began to learn about the tubes in me. They removed my Foley catheter in the morning, and I became mobile. Mary Joy helped me clean up for the day and graciously washed my hair, getting herself wet in the process. Hospital life is not very interesting. However, I had several people call and visit by phone, and of course, Paul and Sharon came to visit in person. I walked around the hospital and proved to everyone that I could move. The day went quickly, and because Paul wanted to get home before the Houston traffic got too bad, they all left about four. Mary Joy left me for the first time in thirty-six hours. I know that she had to have been exhausted. I was perfectly cognizant of my surroundings and of my body now and was doing fine on pain pills. My morphine drip was gone. I could move about. Tuesday night was uneventful, and I rested well.

Saying Good-bye to My Doctor Daughter

Wednesday morning at six, Mary Joy arrived for her final visit. We spent nearly three hours visiting. It was at this point that she told me that she thought that I had thought that I was going to die during this surgery. She and I are very close, and I am very lucky to have her in my life. We were both thankful that the surgery was over and that at least the first news was very good. I was so very thankful that she had come to be with me. She left about 9:00 a.m. to drive back to DFW, where she caught a plane on to her home and work in Detroit.

Son Jeff helped out by taking Sharon to the Hobby Airport, where she caught a noontime flight to Midland, Texas. I had really enjoyed the time that we had shared together also. Sharon and I had been like sisters many years ago. Our lives kind of went separate ways as our families were growing. But now, we had agreed to visit more often and to renew those old bonds. Everyone had left me by midmorning. I was alone in the hospital. Paul was off taking training classes on how to care for my central line and doing business. I decided that I had better get myself going that day and began by getting up to take a bath. It was a little hard getting up and into the bathroom by myself that morning. I hadn't realized before now that I was a little handicapped. I couldn't even reach around far enough to take off the bandages under my arms. I couldn't hold my two cantaloupe-sized drain bulbs and wash myself at the same time.

Seeing My Mastectomy Sites

In the normal process of cleaning up that morning, I took off my gown and looked at myself in the mirror. The person I saw was a bit of a fright. I had swollen red flabs of skin that hanged down under my arms. I had a red cut that ran the whole way across my chest and to my back under each arm. The cut was swollen and uneven. My ribs stuck out farther than my flat sunken chest. My skin around the long incision was red and loose and ugly. My chest looked very ugly to me, and I cried. However, there wasn't a single thing to do about the way that I looked now. My Cancer was gone, and I hoped that I could live over the way that my chest looked. I was not going to wallow in a pity pot so I dried my eyes and decided that I must just go on with my life. I had *to remember the important things.*

After I got over the shock of seeing my new chest without my breasts, I rang the bell to get the nurse in to help me shower. With her help, I took my shower and put on a clean gown. I didn't need to look at my body in the mirror again. I had hopes that it would be better tomorrow. I went back to my bed to hide and to rest.

Talking to the Anesthesiologist about My Nightmares

I got to have my requested talk with the anesthesiologist about my "wake-up experience," and she determined that the dosage of Benadryl that they gave all patients who were receiving the blue sentinel node biopsy dye could cause hallucinations. She and I both felt that this was the culprit. She was sorry that she hadn't realized what was happening to me so that she could have given me medicine to counteract these horrible nightmares that I had lived through. However, she said that she didn't know that I was having them. I wished that I would have been able to contact her in the recovery room. At least now, she knows that this can happen, and maybe she will be more careful in the future.

Laughter Enters My Hospital Room

That day, Paul had to attend two classes to learn how to care for my central line. This apparatus was very important and critical to my well-being through the long process of chemotherapy that was ahead of me. This central line would only work if it was cared for daily *very* carefully. It was a plastic tube that went into my chest and then on down into a big blood vessel. It would be the place where I would receive chemo. Paul attended two classes of one and a half hours each in order to learn the necessary techniques. And after he attended the classes, he had to demonstrate his skills by changing the bandaging on this central line on me for real. He and a Philippine "sergeant nurse" appeared shortly after lunch with bandage packages, and they started the process.

This lady really looked and acted like one of the army nurses in the musical *South Pacific* who controlled everything. She came in and was evidently immediately in charge. She automatically told Paul how to do things. Paul, of course, was a good student. He had taken the instruction class twice and had even taken some notes during the class. He had bought the videotape to take home so that he could review the process. Paul is a smart man, but it didn't take but a few minutes for the nurse to let Paul know that he wasn't "up to snuff" in her books when it came to changing my central line bandage.

The first thing in this process you had to do was to go in and to wash your hands. Paul went in to my bathroom and was busy washing and washing his hands just like he thought that he was supposed to when the nurse told him to hurry up. She hollered, "You can't hide in the bathroom forever." He immediately hollered back, "The instructor told the class attendees that they should wash their hands for thirty seconds very carefully before they began." She replied rather harshly, "This direction has changed now, and fifteen seconds is the acceptable time to wash. Come out and get started on the work." I knew immediately that an interesting show was ahead because Paul is not used to being ordered around, and I lay back to watch it.

Paul came out of the bathroom and with a couple of instructive comments from the sergeant (the nurse), he figured out how to open the bandage package (a small sandwich-size baggie with a covered tray inside). The sergeant had very definite ideas about how everything should be done. Paul had to guardedly take the wrapped-up container out on the table and set it down. He then had to cautiously unfold the disposable and sterilized cloth on the table, revealing a tray with a package of sterilized gloves on top. Next Paul had to carefully lift off and unfold the packages of gloves. Every step he had to do exactly the way that she told him to (which, of course, was not his natural way). She freely and often corrected him and forced him to do it the "right" way. Paul bristled a little but swallowed his pride and continued on.

He had to pick up the right-hand glove with his left hand and to put it on his right hand by only touching the wrist part of the glove. He had to be very careful not to compromise the sterility of everything. The putting on of the gloves was difficult, but he did accomplish it after several strong repeated instructions from the sergeant. He then had to unpack the little carton that contained all of his equipment, and he had to drop the top of the carton without touching his glove to the table. The sergeant wasn't shy about hollering if he looked like he was going to touch his sterile glove to his shirt on his belly or to anything else. I thought that Paul was going to explode a couple of times, but he didn't. Paul is a "take charge" kind of man, one who isn't accustomed to being yelled at on how to do little things.

Paul managed to get everything unpacked from the carton and spread out on the cloth while still keeping his gloves sterile. He was then ready to pick up the scissors and to begin the big work. If I would have been sleepy, I would have had time for a nap during this set-up work, but I was torn between laughing at and feeling sorry for Paul. I had never seen him try so hard to do something that was so unnatural for him for so difficult an instructor. He was ready to go to work now, however. He picked up the scissors, and all of a sudden, I heard the nurse holler again, "Oh, you've done it now. You have touched your scissors to your shirt. You have ruined the sterility of the whole package. We have to start all over. [Grumble, grumble, grumble.]" And she proceeded to grab everything off of the table and to wrap it all back up in the cloth and to throw it into the trash. She then went out of the room with a look of resignation on her face and brought back in another bandaging package. Paul had to start all over again.

I just lay there quietly. I didn't say a word; I just watched. I thought that maybe Paul would explode from his built-up inner anger and might refuse to do this nitpicking job at all, but he didn't. He quietly went into the bathroom to wash his hands again for only fifteen seconds this time. He came back and went through the drill a second time. She hollered several times again, but Paul managed to get the gloves on and the package spread out again. This time, he was more careful with the scissors. She was the ever-watching hawk ready to pounce on him at any incorrect move. It would have been hilarious if it hadn't been so serious. It was my body that we were working on. Paul managed to complete the bandage change and antiseptic washes from this point with only a few near screams from the nurse. We were both relieved when the task was accomplished.

Paul learned to change my bandaging and was an excellent "nurse" for me in this area. He had to swallow his pride and his usual ways of being the authority in order to follow this lady's gruff teaching. He did this because he loved me enough. I am very lucky. I think now that Paul may even laugh someday at the antics that occurred when he took his practical central line training. I know the training certainly livened my day.

Going Home to Spring

After finishing this formidable training task, Paul and I left the hospital and said our good-byes to the wonderful staff at MD Anderson about 3:30 p.m. The trip, although it was really short, only an hour, was difficult. We were in our big red truck that was very bouncy and bumpy. I should have lain down. I hadn't realized at the beginning that the ride would bother me. After we got started, it was difficult to get off of the freeway so that we could stop for me to move to the backseat, where I could lie down. I was greatly distressed by the time that we arrived at Jeff's house. I went inside immediately. The day had been too full, and I was weak, exhausted, and very sore.

Jeff and Liz were fabulous to open their home to us and to help in caring for me. Paul, as always, was my lifeline. He stayed with me constantly and cared for me night and day. My surgery and hospital stay had ended. I knew that I would begin to feel better very soon, and I felt that I would have a life tomorrow. My life would be different, but I hoped that it would be happy. *I knew that I always had to remember the important things in life—love, health, family, and friends.*

Chapter 24

THE REAL BOTTOM

Recovery

Recovery continued. Each day, I got stronger and the pains lessened. I was certainly glad that I had strong pain pills. I had never had a surgery before where I had taken pain pills regularly for any length of time. However, this surgery recovery had proceeded easier, I think, because Paul had been the manager of the pain pills, which I was still taking every four to six hours. My chest burned, and my imaginary boobies hurt when I was off of the pain pills for very long. I was surprised that I was operating so well while I was taking the pain drugs. I had a very long cut that stretched from behind one arm across my chest to behind the other arm. I felt like I had a very tight tiny bra on, and to this day my chest still feels like I am wearing a bra all of the time.

After the surgery, the cut was taped on top and there were no other bandages on me except around my drain spots. Under each arm, I had two holes with two plastic drain tubes coming out of each hole. These four drain tubes went to two big plastic bulbs that hung down below my waist. I didn't have anything to pin the big drain bags to when I got out of bed. The bags were large, about the size of small cantaloupes. I had to send Paul out to the store to buy a big shirt that would cover the ugly things. It took Paul and I over an hour each morning to get me up and "cared for." We had to clean up and empty the drains twice a day. We had to flush the central line daily. I also showered each day. What a big job getting up was, but Paul handled it all very well and never complained. He was very patient, and I tried to also be patient. Some of the tasks were hard for him with his big masculine hands, but he somehow learned to do them anyway. Cancer is a *hard, hard* disease, but now I hoped that it was all out of my body finally.

My daily schedule at this time looked something like this:

- Get up and eat breakfast.
- Go for a walk before it got too awfully hot. (We were in Houston in September.)
- With Paul's help, take my shower.
- Paul will then dress my underarm drain holes and measure and record the drainage.
- Paul will then take care of my central line (or central venous catheter) that require a complete dressing change twice a week and a daily heparin shot (a blood thinner to keep the CVC line open).
- I then take another pain pill, rest, and/or nap until lunch.
- Eat lunch.
- Take another rest and/or nap.
- About 3:45 p.m., when Erica comes home from school, I visit with her for a while.
- Eat supper.
- Watch a movie or TV or visit with the family.
- Before bed, Paul has to change the dressings on my underarm drain holes and measure and record the drainage.
- Take another pain pill and go to bed for the night. I was regular in waking up during the night about every four hours so that I could take another pain pill. My chest pain was a good alarm clock.

A Bump in the Road

We hit a bump in the road Saturday, September 20. The day before had just not been good for me. The left side of my body got so sore on Friday night that I could no longer lie on it. I had the end of the surgical cut and two drain holes under my arm on each side, but before this night, I had been able to lie on both sides. Saturday morning, I woke up with fever. I had at least a couple of degrees of fever all day. We called the MD Anderson help numbers Saturday morning, reporting my condition in messages. By Saturday afternoon, when we had not gotten a callback, Paul called again. This time, he spoke to a person who had the surgeon-on-call call us back. He, of course, told us that he would have to see me to know what to do. He did tell us that Dr. Ralston's Fellow was on duty at the hospital that weekend. Paul and I hung up the phone and then set about to decide whether to drive down to MD Anderson or not.

We went upstairs and took the bandage off of the drain holes under the left arm. The redness around the drain holes had increased to be about three inches in diameter. In the morning, the redness had only been about the size of a quarter. We both looked at the increased red circle and agreed that we needed to go to the ER. Fortunately, we were in Spring, Texas, which is a northern suburb of Houston. It was only about a forty-five-minute drive to the ER at MD Anderson.

We took Jeff's sedan (not our big red pickup which was so rough for me to ride in at this time) and drove to MD Anderson. We arrived about 4:45 p.m., and I was in a bed there by 5:40 p.m. The ER nurse saw me quickly, looked things over, and ordered blood tests, a urine test, and an IV. She paged the surgeon on call, Dr. Ralston's Fellow. My nurse came in and started laying out seven little tubes for blood. He brought in an IV pole with bags of water and an antibiotic on it. He happily told me that he was going to do all of the work without ever even sticking me. I was amazed. I had blood drawn, took an IV, and didn't get a single needle stick. The nurse used the central line to do everything. I thought that evening that maybe this central line wouldn't be so bad after all.

The Surgical Fellow arrived and took off the bandages on my left side. She cleaned the long surgical cut with iodine and reapplied the bandages. To my surprise, when the doctor first took off the bandages on this long cut, my chest didn't pop open. I complained about the "tight-rope feeling" around my chest where the cut was, and she explained that the feeling was normal. I guessed then that over time, it would either go away or I would get used to it. She proceeded to clean all of my cuts, gave me a prescription for Augmentin (850 mg), and dismissed me. Paul and I were glad that we were able to catch this infection early in the cycle. We were glad that we were still in Houston.

The Good News Comes

On Tuesday, September 23, we received the call from Dr. Ralston's PA on the pathology report from my surgery. I was amazed to find out that there was absolutely *no cancer* found in any of the tissue taken in my surgery. They had taken out five more lymph nodes from under my right arm. None of them contained Cancer. They took off the right breast. It did not have any of the invasive carcinoma Cancer in it. That means that on July 21, when Dr. Dover did my second lumpectomy in Durango, or on August 14, when Dr. Ralston did my clean-out surgery at MD Anderson, one of them removed all of the Cancer. The tissue from my left breast showed no Cancer. Dr. Ralston had removed one sentinel node and one backup lymph node from under my left arm and both of these were negative for Cancer. What a *wonderful* prognosis! No Cancer was found from this surgery.

We were, of course, ecstatic with the good news. My prayer/support group had done a miraculous job. Someone in the group must have had a direct line to God and worked overtime talking to him about me. This report was exactly what I had been asking for in my prayers. I was very thankful and happy.

I now felt like I was at the bottom of the awful black monster-filled pit. *When you reach the bottom of the hole, there is no way to go but up.* I could now start the climb back up to the light and the real world again. The worst had passed. I had made it through the darkest part of the night. I couldn't see the dawning yet, but I knew that it was ahead. That awful Cancer in its organized form was now all *out of my body*! There still might be pilgrim cells of the Cancer that were sent out from the main colony, but the main colony and all of its immediate support had been removed.

Chapter 25

Don't Go It Alone

Returning Home

Paul and I left Houston on Wednesday, September 24, to return to our Grapevine home. The trip was long. I slept in the backseat nearly the whole way. I was tired when we arrived, but I was also excited to be home.

Mr. Boots, my cat, seemed very happy to see us and sat in my lap for over an hour that night. He sat in my lap, put his front feet up on the lower part of my chest, and looked right at my chin and my flat chest. He didn't step up on my sore chest. He looked at me like he knew that I had been hurt and that he wanted to give me a kiss, but he and I are kind of formal with each other, so he just looked politely. He did stay with me and slept peacefully on my lap all the time that I sat in my chair that evening. He was very loving and comforting to me that Wednesday evening.

I walked each day. I had lost a little weight. I was getting stronger each day. I still needed my pain pills, however, but I was hopeful that next week, the cuts would be well enough for me to taper off of the pain pills. I was actually functioning okay on the pain pills, which was a surprise to me. I still had my two small cantaloupe-sized drains hanging on each side. They looked yucky, but I was actually getting used to having them. I had figured out how to hold them in my hand or else in between my knees when I showered. Paul no longer had to stand there getting wet holding them while I showered. Paul was becoming an efficient nurse, and he had always been a meticulous caregiver. What would I have done without him?

Another Setback

I finished taking the additional dose of the powerful antibiotic, Augmentin (875 mg), on Tuesday, September 30. The doctor had prescribed this for me when the drain cut under my right arm had gotten infected six days after my double mastectomy. On Wednesday, October 1, just after lunch, I became very sick. I went to bed and began to get the shakes and the chills. The chill shakings became so violent that I thought that I was having seizures. Paul took my temperature, and it was 102.6 degrees. He immediately called MD Anderson and reached Dr. Ralston Physican's Assistant (PA). Paul described my condition, and she told him to get me to the emergency room in Grapevine immediately. We left immediately to go to the hospital, and I checked in to the ER at 3:45 p.m.

I went in to see the triage nurse after only a short wait. When I told her that my temperature was 102.6, she immediately took me back to a bed even though the ER waiting room was full of people. When the nurse took my temperature, my fever in the last half hour had gone up to 103.8. I saw the ER doctor shortly after 4:00 p.m. Remember that in our last trip to the ER at this hospital, when my boob had exploded in the night, we had waited hours and hours before we saw the doctor. With this incident, I had three doctors at my bedside very quickly. Of course, this incident occurred on a Wednesday afternoon before 5:00 p.m. and the visit to the ER with the burst boob had occurred about midnight on a Friday night. Working on my case was a surgeon, an internist, and the ER doctor.

I received an IV of fluids, Tylenol, Motrin, and drip antibiotics immediately. Of course, nothing that I took in my by mouth stayed down in my tummy. I was nauseated and threw up anything that I swallowed. They ordered x-rays, blood tests, and a sonogram; gathered my medical history verbally and by copying my medical notebook, which we remembered to grab as we ran out of the door at our house; and held conferences. They suspected that my central line (CVC) was the source of the infection to cause the high fever.

We called my two sons, John Hyde and Paul Damian Hyde, who lived in the Dallas/Fort Worth metroplex area. And of course, I called my doctor daughter, Mary Joy. John and Paul Damian and his wife Stephanie immediately came to the ER to be with me.

After a little while in the ER, my temperature changed directions and began to go down a little. By the time that I got up to my hospital room at 8:00 p.m., I was feeling much better. The first thing that the nurse did when I got to my room was to pull out my central line. They carefully put the tip of the catheter from the central line into a sterile bottle to be sent off to the lab to be cultured for bacteria. I hated to have this line pulled since I would have to go through another surgery to get it put in again. However, the doctors and even Mary Joy thought that the central line was the source of the infection since my surgery cuts looked like they were healing normally. My central line did not look like it was infected, but I could not second-guess my doctors.

Now I would have to do all of the medical injections the old-fashioned way—using a needle in my arm. My left wrist and hand soon turned black and blue from the many blood draws that were done during this hospital stay. My veins in my left arm seemed to just shrink and disappear when they saw someone coming with a needle. Because I had had all of the lymph nodes removed from under my right arm, I would never be able to receive shots or needle sticks of any kind in the right limb. No one could take my blood pressure on the right arm either. We always had to watch to be sure that these rules (no pressure or no sticks to the right arm) were observed. I needed to purchase a medical alert bracelet that I would always wear, making medical personnel aware of my situation. Since I still had big drains hanging off of me, everyone knew that I had recently had some important surgeries.

About 10:00 p.m., Paul Damian Stephanie, John, and Paul all left the hospital for the night. I was alone to face the ravages and the damage that this Cancer monster had left in my body. It was very dark outside, and I could not see the stars. I wondered what lay ahead for me in this big battle. I had successfully finally gotten the immediate Cancer out of my body, but now I had more health issues to face. I was not as scared as I had been during the first part of this fight. I felt that I surely could fight and win over the health problems that arose as an aside from the Cancer. I had been so healthy and strong just a few months ago. I had no idea why this was happening to me. My thoughts wound down, and I soon settled into peaceful conditions that led to sleep. Before dropping off, *I resolved that I had better get my prayer support team and all my friends engaged.* I knew that I would need all of their help again, and with this help, I knew that I would fight longer, facing each new battle as it happened.

The Hospital Again

I spent the first days in my room in the Baylor Hospital in Grapevine, Texas, just enduring lots of blood tests, often three a day. The doctors had no idea what "bug" had caused my fever and therefore could not prescribe the correct medicine to fight it. Every day, we all worked to keep my temperature down close to normal. I received an IV fluid bag and an antibiotic bag continuously. When my temperature went up even slightly, I began to get this overall bad feeling. It was almost like someone just took a paintbrush and colored my whole body black. I didn't hurt in any specific place, but I just felt *bad*.

Paul, as the good caregiver that he was, would always ask me how I felt and where I hurt. He had trouble understanding when I told him that "I just felt bad." I cried and got very depressed when I felt "bad." My real physical pain seemed to be magnified at these times, and I spiraled down into a "depression hole." We had experienced these same feelings and problems earlier after my surgeries. From this hospital experience where fever was really the only symptom that we fought, I decided that low-grade fevers had been the cause of my bad feelings before. We vowed to watch my temperature carefully in the future. To help my feelings, at the high recommendation of the triage nurse in the ER, the doctor prescribed an antidepressant for me.

I couldn't imagine taking this kind of medicine. I had always been in charge and in control of my life. I had never needed a crutch medicine to get me through, but I found out that I did need it this time.

I also found out that I had to work really hard to learn how to read my body and to be able to recognize when I was starting to crash physically and psychologically. I underwent a CT scan of the lower abdomen. My liver enzymes were high when I entered the hospital, so more evaluations on my liver were done. The doctors decided that the long use of the pain medication with a high dosage of Tylenol caused me to have liver problems. My pain medication was switched to a pill that contained high doses of aspirin. I was impatient to go home. I was ready to get on with my battle against Cancer. I was missing my scheduled appointments at MD Anderson.

As the days dragged by, the surgeon decided that my mastectomy surgery had not been the cause of the infection, so he left the case. The internist from my doctor's group turned me over to the hospital doctor. This hospital doctor called in the infectious disease doctor to join the team, and they finally determined that I had two bad types of bacteria in my blood. The worst of these was a gram-negative bacterium, which usually came from the GI tract or perhaps from a central line. It appeared at this time that the infection may have come with the central line. The good news that we received when the blood cultures finally identified the "bugs" that I had was that they were treatable with pill antibiotics. A lot of the bad bugs must be treated with IV antibiotics. By being able to take the antibiotic in a pill meant that I could go back home. I left the hospital on Monday, October 6, five days after I had entered.

I had only planned to give one year of my life to Cancer. I had vowed to myself that I would have this battle over and done with by June 2004. I was pushing really hard to be able to meet this deadline, but there were so many things that I just couldn't control that kept slowing things down. This third emergency only emphasized the point that we needed to get down to Houston and stay there so that I could always be treated by my own doctors. I couldn't believe that we got caught in the Grapevine ER a second time! I thought that we had learned that lesson *(stay in the same area with your doctors)*, but I guess that we hadn't. I felt that our next trip to Houston would include finding an apartment. I now expected to spend the winter in Houston. We would only visit some weekends back in Grapevine. We knew that we needed to have our residence close to the place where I was undergoing Cancer treatments.

My surgery cut continued to heal. Some of the pieces of sterile tapes were falling off, and I began to think that the scar was going to be small eventually. I still had the awful huge drains hanging from under my arms. I would feel a lot better if I could get rid of them. I wrote the following to my support people while I was in the hospital:

I guess that we should not ever stop praying. I had indicated that I was doing fine, but then this monster Cancer rose up and bit me again out of the clear blue. This is the toughest disease that I have ever had. I hope that I never have to fight this battle ever again. I pray that I will not die from Cancer. I might die from falling from a beautiful cliff in Colorado, or maybe I will just die peacefully in my sleep some night. I think that dying from an illness will just be too hard. The couple that owned our Colorado house before us had a strange and sad story that comes to my mind at this time. The wife had breast Cancer and committed suicide by jumping from a moving car about a year before we bought the house. I had wondered how in the world that she could ever do something like that, but now I think I understand how she might have come to that decision. However, I am not sure that I would be strong enough to die from Cancer. I will beat this Cancer. My disease is curable. I will take the treatments that the best doctors that I can find recommend. I will walk the path and suffer the pain and the weakness, knowing that on the other side of this road is life and health. Again let me thank each of you for your help and support. Not a single day goes by without someone sending a card, an e-mail, a telephone call, or something that lets me know that others are thinking about me and pulling for me. I know that God is in charge and that everything will be okay in the end. Thank you for sharing my burden. I just don't think I am strong enough to travel this road by myself.

Chapter 26

Hard Times Are Relative—
Remember Job from the Bible?

Home Again from the Hospital

On Monday, October 6, I was released from the hospital, armed with another big dose of a special antibiotic meant to kill the bad bugs that had somehow gotten into my body with my last surgery, the double mastectomy. I was very glad to get back into my own environment, but I was awfully weak. In the hospital, the "mode" was to stay in bed. At home, the opposite was true, and it was very apparent that I had to stay in bed most of the time until my strength returned. I would be up for a couple of hours, and then I had to go back to bed. However, I got stronger each day. The mornings were the best. I still saved a pain pill to take in the late afternoons. Although several mornings included a nice nap after breakfast, I generally got any real work done that I did for the day completed in the morning.

The weather in Texas was really nice. The temperatures had cooled into the high seventies and low eighties in the day times. At least some of the time, we had low humidities. The trees were beginning to yellow, and bright yellow and purple mums and Halloween goblins were appearing in the neighborhood yards. Fall was here.

Earlier Hard Times

I had experienced hard times before in my life. I had been involved in a bad car wreck and had suffered a back injury. I suffered from back pain for many months after this wreck. This was a difficult time in my life, as I had four small children to care for and a husband who was gone for many days at a time. It was really hard for me to get my work done in the new peach orchard and to care for my children. However, this bad time passed with no lasting scars on my life.

My first husband worked for Braniff when it declared bankruptcy and closed its doors in the 1970s. We had a very difficult time financially for many years afterward. In fact, my twenty-two-year marriage to this man ended in divorce in 1986. All of these years were very difficult and hard. It wasn't easy to break apart a union that had been so long. I hated this time, but I got through it. I was changed and scarred, but I went on and so did my life.

My Cancer—The Next Hard Time

In June, 2003, I entered my Cancer period. You have read of the "hard times" that I had come through thus far in the unplanned journey. I truly believe that this was the most difficult "hard time" that I had ever experienced. It was a time of pain, blood, narcotic medicines, high-powered antibiotics of all forms, bandages, catheters that remained in my body for months, swelling, fever, IV bottles, needles, nurses (both good and poor), doctors whom you depended on, x-rays, CT scans, wheelchairs, beds, uncertainties, and fears. There seemed to be no end to the new things that I had to face. At this time, October, 2003, I reeled from the havoc that the Cancer double mastectomy surgery had wreaked on my body. However, I sincerely hoped that this "hard time" like all of my others would pass, and I hoped to return to a normal life, scarred but well. *Looking back on the earlier "hard times" in my life, I could see that they weren't really as bad as I had thought.*

Another Crisis

Finally, the drainage numbers that we carefully measured several times a day as we changed and cleaned the drainage bulbs that hung from under my arms fell below thirty milliliters in each bulb for a twenty-four-hour period. I had the four tubes pulled from under my arms on Thursday, October 9. I was so happy to get those things removed. Three and a half weeks after surgery was long enough to worry with those foreign apparatuses.

However, Saturday, October 11, late in the afternoon, I began to feel sick again. I took a pain pill at 5:00 p.m. and started to feel a little better by 6:00 p.m. When I lay down in bed at 8:00 p.m., I happened to put my hand up on my chest where the surgery cut was, just to feel my chest like I often did. I felt soft, moving, swollen flesh. My surgical area was storing fluid and was swelling. I showed Paul, and I began to think of making another trip to Houston. I did not want to have another emergency at the Grapevine Hospital. All kinds of thoughts ran through my mind. Would the fluid cause the stitches to bust? Could my body absorb this fluid before its quantities became damaging to my skin? Would it be painful again? How would I face another crisis?

Since it was 10:00 p.m. on a Saturday night, there wasn't a lot of medical help around, Paul and I finally just went to sleep. He had to sleep and to rest if we were going to drive to Houston on Sunday. Murphy's Law says that if something can go wrong, it will. I began to think that this one law was ruling my life. I just couldn't seem to find a time when something difficult did not happen.

My Job Time

I thought that this Cancer time was perhaps my *Job* period. Job being the Biblical character in the Old Testament that God allowed the Devil to test. When I was getting my bachelor's degree in the early 1960s, one of my English class term papers was a study of the book of Job. I remembered reading and rereading this famous and often overlooked Biblical treatise. Job was a wonderful man of God. He was a good servant of God and was very prosperous. However, the Devil and God got into a conversation about Job, and the Devil said that Job was only good because he was so prosperous. The Devil said that Job would surely deny God if he wasn't so rich. God felt that this was not the case and allowed the devil to test Job. Job, who at the beginning of the book was rich with wives and many children and lots of livestock, lost everything in this test. But still Job praised God.

The devil came back to God again and told the Lord that Job remained a servant of God because his body was healthy and strong. So God allowed the Devil to attack Job's physical body, and Job got sick with awful sores all over his body. He nearly died, but Job did *not* renounce his God. This was a very bleak and black time in Job's life. I thought that this time was a bleak and black time in my life also. I was scared that something was really wrong with my surgery since my underarms were swelling so much. I certainly had not suffered like Job, but for me, who had lived a "charmed" life before Cancer, it made me ask if I was being tested. I wondered if God was allowing the Devil to try my soul and my faith. I hoped that the nightmare that Cancer brought would end soon and the final chapter of Job would apply to me. In the last few chapters of the book of Job, God restored Job's life even richer than it had been before the Devil scourged him. The book had a "and he lived happily ever after" ending. That ending was very comforting to me.

This weekend, when my body was swelling, I couldn't imagine what was wrong, I imagined all kinds of terrible things happening.

My Fluid Collection

That Sunday morning, my fluid swellings were not larger. Paul thought that my increased activities on Saturday—attending a few garage sales for a couple of hours, driving the car around, and lifting a few things—might have caused the buildup of fluid. I hoped that his diagnosis was correct. I prayed that my body would be able to absorb the fluid and that the buildup would not increase. I planned to rest throughout the day. I was not going out. I would have loved to have gone to church, but I knew that I would have just cried there. If someone asked me how I was doing, I might have felt the need to tell him or her how I really felt and that would undo me for sure. I wrote in my newsletter at that time the following:

> I am certain that this adventure will end happily and that I will be a little scarred, a lot wiser, and more appreciative of life's little blessings. However, right now, the path isn't easy. The Cancer growths are all gone from my body, but the monster continues to attack. Pray for me. Thank you very much for traveling this road with me.

After my rest on Sunday, the swelling did not seem to increase. We decided that we would drive to Houston on Monday and go to MD Anderson on Tuesday morning. There just never seemed to be an end to this battle.

Back to MD Anderson

On Tuesday, October 14, we returned to MD Anderson and my surgeon's PA drained the fluid from under my right arm. She used a four-inch-diameter gathering bottle and a big needle that she stuck into the fluid sack around my scar. She took out about one-half to three-fourths inch (60 cc) of clear yellow fluid, measured in the gathering bottle. She stuck me about three more times in different places with the needle but could not get out much more fluid because the fluid had separated into different pockets. She explained that this fluid draining was not abnormal. The surgery cut and the resulting cavity was so large that there would be fluid production for some time after the wound on the outside healed. Since I had no lymph nodes under my right arm that would normally absorb this fluid, my body had to learn a new way to send this fluid to other lymph nodes in my body to finally be absorbed. She opted not to drain any of the fluid from under my left arm. My left arm was collecting fluid also (not as much), but my left side had a nearly intact lymph system and should be able to handle the fluid.

The PA said that eventually I would be able to stop getting this fluid drained from the outside. Surprisingly, it hadn't hurt for her to stick that big needle into my skin. My skin around the surgical site was completely numb. When I put down my arms after the draining, I felt the full pouches under my left arm while my right arm rested flat against my body. However, everything felt better. I had her check and drain my right underarm again before we left Houston to return to Grapevine.

Early on Wednesday morning, October 15, from Houston, I wrote in one of my medical updates the following optimistic words:

> I am really getting better now! I am going to get well soon! In the mornings, I actually feel good. My surgery cut is still tight, but it doesn't hurt in the mornings. I know that each day, I will feel better longer and longer until soon, I will be well from this awful surgery. The Cancer monster has made this one of the most difficult surgeries that I have ever had.

Chapter 27

GETTING READY FOR CHEMOTHERAPY

Finding Out about My Chemo

I finally met with my oncologist, Dr. Brawn. Even though he had that name, he fussed at me because I had put down on an entrance questionnaire that I had six drinks per week. I assured him that I was drinking *nothing* since I started this Cancer routine. He seemed nice and was very knowledgeable. He talked really fast so I had to listen quickly to catch all that he was saying. He explained that I would be receiving about six months of chemotherapy. The MD Anderson standard concoction for me was Taxol and FAC which is a composition of 5-Fu (Flourouracil), Adraimycin, Cytoxan.

My chemo treatments would be divided into two different treatment regimens. In the first treatment phase, I would receive Taxol that would be given in two—to three-hour IV treatments on one day each week for twelve weeks. In the second treatment phase, I would receive FAC for three days, one time every three weeks. I was to repeat this series four times. A central line catheter would be required for this second phase of chemo. The chemo in this phase would be delivered through an IV, and because the treatment would continue for forty-eight hours, I would wear a backpack pump all but the first few hours of this time so that the FAC would drip into my body. Then I would rest for a number of days and repeat this treatment 21 days later.

My Chances of Getting Breast Cancer Again

While we were with my oncologist, we asked him about the chances of my getting Cancer again. Figuring the probabilities of my Cancer ever returning was really a statistical nightmare, but Dr. Brawn had been asked this question many times before. He pulled out his charts and gave me the following facts for a stage 2 Cancer like I had:

Women over fifty who have some kind of chemotherapy reduce their risk of reoccurrence of the breast Cancer (which is about 50 percent) by a third. FAC reduces the reoccurrence by 50 percent more. Taking Tamoxofin after you finish the chemotherapy reduces the reoccurrence further by 47 percent. Anyway, when I finish my chemo, I think that I will have only about a 15 percent chance of this Cancer reoccurring elsewhere in my body.

Without breasts, I will be done with breast Cancer for a lifetime, I hope. That is my fervent prayer anyway.

American Cancer Society Help

After a nice lunch at the hospital cafeteria, I met with several other women who had recently undergone mastectomies. The volunteer who lead the meeting was representing the American Cancer Society in the "Reach for Recovery" program. She had undergone a mastectomy herself several years ago so she knew what she was talking about. She gave each of us in the class a bra (of the size that we requested) with a simple prosthesis (a boob thing of cloth that she filled with polyester stuffing). I had never gotten to choose the size of the boobs that I wanted before. I discovered now that I could easily do that. She answered all of our questions, and we watched a video showing us the exercises that we should do to get the movement back in our arms. I use the plural in all of these references because I had a double mastectomy. Both of my arms were affected. It was a good thing to talk with her.

I was eligible to participate in a new chemotherapy study using a new drug. After discussing this study with Dr. Brawn and my doctor daughter, we decided to *not* participate in the study. I began my chemo treatments on Monday, October 27. I had a chemo treatment on each of eleven Mondays following this date.

Chemotherapy "How To" Class

In the late afternoon, I attended the required chemo "how to" class. The class was very informative. Paul and I both attended and first watched a video that gave us an overview of the side effects of chemotherapy and how to treat them. An experienced Breast Center nurse led the class. She answered our questions and gave us tips about what to do and what not to do while I was in chemotherapy. I also was given a manual with all of the information on the side effects of chemo, my "How To Manual" for the next six months. This ended our long day at MD Anderson.

Moving to Houston

The next day, Thursday, October 16, we went apartment hunting. We looked at six different apartment complexes. We chose the Gates at Hermann Park Apartments. Our apartment was on the ground floor and had a small patio that opened up to a rather long but narrow grassed and fenced area for the whole building. I thought that Mr. Boots, my kitty, would think that it was his own private backyard.

Moving to Houston and renting an unfurnished apartment meant that we would have to purchase some furniture. I wanted to buy a new king-size mattress and box springs. We needed this larger mattress in our home in Grapevine anyway. I had gone to garage sales in Houston and had bought a lot of used furniture and other things. I was very frugal with my purchases and made Paul's money go a long ways. We stored my purchases in Jeff's garage in Spring.

We drove to Grapevine Saturday afternoon. It had been a busy but fruitful time in Houston. We then spent three days getting packed and taking care of our house arrangements so that we could leave it for a long period of time. Paul took care of business and his health matters, and we packed our Toyota Camry sedan and our big red pickup. We really didn't take too much furniture with us. We brought lots of boxes of "stuff" (kitchen equipment, food, clothes, and miscellaneous supplies). We had the pickup completely loaded. My car was full also. I was able to go to our Grapevine church, Living Word, one last time and had said my good-byes to our friends.

On Tuesday, October 21, we finished up the last-minute leaving chores, put Mr. Boots into the car, said good-bye to our wonderful neighbors, and left Grapevine in a small caravan. I drove the Toyota Camry, and Paul drove the big red truck. When we arrived in Houston at our complex, I hired some Mexican workers at the apartment complex to unload our cars. Paul and our son, Jeff, went to Costco's to purchase our new king-size mattress and box springs. I started unpacking in our new home.

When we finally got settled into our messy new apartment with a bed, it was 9:00 p.m. Mr. Boots sat in my lap again for a long, long time. We only had one chair, the vibrating massage chair, and Mr. Boots even sat in my lap while I got a massage. We went to bed exhausted.

I was now in Houston for the duration of the rest of this battle. I was set to take the next big step in ridding my body of any hidden Cancer cells—chemotherapy.

Chapter 28

Taxol Chemo Treatments

Chemo to Begin

Our stay in Houston had begun. We had managed to somehow make the move from Grapevine to Houston quickly and without any more big setbacks in my health. I hadn't felt up to making a move, but with everyone's help, the move was made. The apartment was still a mess when my chemo treatments started, but we were now living just a few blocks from MD Anderson and my doctors. We had decided to start the first treatment on Monday, October 27. We had decided on this day so that we could get through the holidays without me having to take a chemo treatment on Thanksgiving or Christmas.

Settling In

We didn't know many people at this time being new comers to Houston. I immediately began attending some of the programs that MD Anderson offered for its patients. I took advantage of the counselors that MD Anderson provided for each patient and began regular weekly counseling sessions. I had so badly needed this kind of help during the first part of my battle with Cancer, but I just hadn't been in one place long enough to get the counseling going. Now that we had settled for the duration of the unplanned journey, I immediately sought help. My counselor agreed to meet with me each week. Facing a complex and difficult disease causes even very strong people to doubt their abilities and their inner beliefs. I recommend that *if you are facing Cancer, you should seek out counseling help so that you can discuss your private and inner fears and thoughts.* Getting these things out into the open with someone who is caring and knowledgeable really helps.

We went to church that first Sunday, October 26, in Houston at the Lutheran Church on the Rice University Campus. I greatly needed the security and the reinforcement of my religious beliefs that I always get from God's house. I love being a part of a church family. This church was close to our apartment and easy to find.

This church had two features that I really liked. The first feature was its name, Christ the King Lutheran, which was the same name as our home church in Durango. Its second feature was a huge, beautiful pipe organ with great pewter pipes that spread across the front of the building. This organ had real clanging bells that rang from the tall steeple when church started and when it was ending. This church also had a professional organist from Rice University, whose preludes and postludes were concerts in themselves. However, it was a cold church, and we eventually left it even though it was located very close to our apartment.

My First Chemo Treatment

On Monday, October 27, I took my first chemo treatment. I went into the chemo room at 3:30 p.m. and was released about 10:00 p.m. I took three preparation packs of medicines: Benadryl and two bags of antinausea drugs. I then took a two-hour infusion of the Cancer killer, Taxol. One of the preparation packs caused me to have a slight reaction, so the nurse stopped it immediately and flushed the line with saline. She then started the pack again very, very slowly, so my treatment took longer than normal. I was very comfortable, however, and could not stay awake for the whole thing. I ended up sleeping for about one and a half hours during the treatment.

Paul, who was carefully watching me, kept waking me up and asking me how I was doing. I felt a few stomach cramps the next morning and suffered with diarrhea. I felt slightly ill and was a little nauseated. However, I was doing well. I was drinking my two liters of water each day. The nurses advised me to drink lots of water so that my body could flush out the chemo quickly. Everything at the moment seemed fine. I would take these treatments each Monday for the next eleven weeks.

Living with Chemo

The first week after the chemo began was an adventure. I really did not know quite what to expect. I didn't feel really bad. However, when I cut my husband's hair on Friday morning after the chemo treatment on Monday, I developed back pain that was debilitating. I had been in a car wreck many years ago, where I was pinned inside of a car. The lower quadrant of my back was injured at that time. Since then, I sometimes had lower back pain but this pain was different.

I normally cut Paul's hair, so this activity was not a new activity for me. I do stand when I cut, and I have to hold both of my arms up, but the act of cutting is not strenuous in any way. However, after having had the chemo and cutting Paul's hair, I suffered with a painful backache. I called the nurse in the Breast Clinic at MD Anderson, and she told me to take pain medication. Taking one pill did not cut the pain, but when I took a second pill, I got relief. I was always impressed when I was in pain to find how good pain pills made me feel. They were wonder drugs. After hurting pretty badly for a few hours, when I took a pain pill, I got this feeling of well-being and an "almost high" that was fabulous. I always thought that these were the feelings that caused dumb people to get hooked on pain-relieving drugs. When I took them regularly, the normality of them ruined this "high" feeling for me, and all I had left was that "drugged" feeling, which I hated. I guess this saved me from becoming addicted.

Anyway by taking pain medication on Friday afternoon, my back pain was relieved so that by Saturday, I felt normal again. We went to see a Rice football game that beautiful Saturday afternoon. It was a very exciting game, and I enjoyed a "normal" fall acitvity.

After the game, we went out to Peter's (our number two son's) house in Clearwater to celebrate Halloween by joining them that evening as their children went trick or treating in the neighborhood. The weather was nice and warm, and it was a really nice outing for me. The pain pills had made the visit and the walk possible. This was our first real holiday in Houston. We got back to our apartment that evening about 9:00 p.m.

The Halloween fun with the children had been a wonderful diversion from my chemo. Cancer had "taken a powder" from my life and thoughts for a while. My first week of chemo was going to end on a festive note.

On Sunday morning, November 2, before church, I decided that I would clean out a closet that held my BeautiControl products. I needed to fill a customer's order. I set about moving my entire inventory around and straightening out the closet at the same time. Just as I was finishing this task, I felt my back seize. I immediately went over to my very comfortable chair to sit down. I had to take another pain pill. This second time that my back had seized the pain was much worse than it had been the first time. I vowed at this point to be *very* careful and not to lift any more boxes for a while.

Draw a Chart of Your Task Time

The first week of my six months of chemo had passed. To help me get through this time, I made a chart of the days of time that I had to spend doing chemo. I drew lines of two squares all across the page. I put the date of each day and the name of the day of the week in the top square, and I left the square below each date blank. This was a drawing of the time that I planned to spend taking chemo. My homemade, hand drawn chart did not look as neat as the abbreviated computer prepared chart that you see below. However, the principle of the work is the same.

BREAST CANCER: THE UNPLANNED JOURNEY - LESSONS LEARNED

MY CHEMO JOURNEY

October, 2003							November 2003							
Treatment #	1						2							3
Weekday	M	T	W	Th	F	S	S	M	T	W	Th	F	S	S	M
Number	27	28	29	30	31	1	2	3	4	5	6	7	8	9	10
Done	XX	X	X	X	X	X	X	XX	X	X	X	X	X	X	XX

April, 2004														
Treatment #	3				LAST FAC TREATMENT									
Weekday	Th	F	S	S	M	T	W	Th	F	S	S	M	T	W	Th
Number	1	2	3	4	5	6	7	8	9	10	11	12	13	14	15
Done	X	X	X	X	XX	XX	XX	X	X	X	X	X	X	X	X

April, 2004														
Treatment #	4													
Weekday	F	S	S	M	T	W	Th	F	S	S	M	T	W	Th	F
Number	16	17	18	19	20	21	22	23	24	25	26	27	28	29	30
Done	X	X	X	X	X	X	X	X							

Last appointment at MD

Leave Houston for Tx. home

    Charting the time and required tasks of something that you have to do, marking off each day as it passes, and then being able to see one's progress seems to make a long and difficult task easier. I had made a chart similar to this one many years ago when I had a job that I did not like. At that time, I made a chart of weeks that ran for seven years. My new chart only ran for six months. I used magnets to put my Chemo Task Chart up on the refrigerator door, and each evening, I used my big black magic marker to x off each day as it passed. I could look at my chart at any time and see immediately how much time I had left to work through this chemo task. *Quantifying the time involved in finishing a difficult task seems to make it easier to accomplish.* I would advise each Cancer patient to chart his time and then to record his progress. As you get more x's on the chart, you feel a sense of progress and accomplishment.

Chapter 29

Bald and Beautiful

Second Treatment

On Monday, November 3, I took my second chemo treatment. This time, my appointment was at 1:00 p.m., but they were running late, and I didn't get into the bed in the chemo unit until 3:00 p.m. We finished this treatment at 7:00 p.m. The time duration of my Taxol infusion was cut in half. I did not take the third small package of medicine, the steroid. I still had to take the Benadryl at a reduced rate, but our administration time was reduced from seven hours to four hours. I never enjoyed spending my time in the chemo unit.

I had diarrhea again as soon as I got home from my second chemo treatment. Because of that and some vomiting, I was sick Tuesday. I also suffered from extreme soreness in my right elbow joint and in my right knee. I got a prescription filled that the doctor had given me earlier for a medicine that helped me with this new side effect. I was sick again on Thursday. My fever went up on those "sick" days, but the sickness at this point only lasted about twenty-four hours. The difficult thing was that I just didn't know when it would strike.

Third Treatment

On the next Monday, November 10, I went to the hospital and took my third treatment. Everything went normally. Wednesday we drove up to Crockett, Texas, to preview the town for my daughter, Mary Joy. She and her doctor husband, Tarl, were evaluating positions in that small Texas town. In my opinion, Crockett seemed to be a going and moving small town. Making this preview evaluation was a very nice distraction for me. This duty or job took me away from my Cancer battle for a day.

I was forced to get the skin under my right arm drained again on Friday, November 7. The nurse drained out 80 cc of fluid. I really wished that this fluid buildup would stop. However, it had been two weeks since it had been drained before so at least the fluid collection was going longer now between drainings. Not having any lymph nodes on my right side looked now to be a real handicap.

Sunday I got to visit with my doctor daughter, Mary Joy. We met her and her husband at the Houston airport. It was really nice to see them. She looked very pretty. We caught up on the news, looked at the houses that they were reviewing in Crockett, and hugged a bunch. I thought that they would probably sign the contracts for their jobs in Crockett. Much too soon, our airport visit was over. It was time for them to leave to catch their flight back to their work in Detroit, Michigan. Mary Joy is a sweet and wonderful daughter, and I am very lucky to have her. Family support is so very important during your Cancer fight. *Be with your family for pleasant times as much as you can.* Seeing Mary Joy that Sunday afternoon buoyed my spirits so that the next day's chemo treatment was easier.

Passing the Time between Treatments

Quickly we discovered that going to the movies was a great way to spend available afternoons between my Taxol treatments. We enjoyed these shows, and even during chemo, when I was weak and not feeling so good, this entertainment still worked wonders on my spirit by helping me forget my real-world troubles. I could go to the movies even when I felt tired and sore. I couldn't go when I was nauseated or had diarrhea. When I was weak, Paul would drop me at the front door to the movie theater while he parked the car. I always had the strength to make it into the dark theater seat and to enjoy the "make believe" world of someone.

I was walking at this time as much as I could. I walked two miles when I went to MD Anderson and back. I walked to the hospital again on Tuesday but had to call Paul to come get me to get home because I didn't have the strength to make the return trip. Paul and I sometimes walked around our block, which was quite a long walk. I hoped that when it got cooler, I could walk more. I knew that I needed the exercise, but some days it was really hard to find the energy to do much at all.

Thoughts about Chemo from My Letters

One often feels very discouraged during a chemo battle. Even having had only three treatments, I still felt awful at times. The following is another excerpt from one of the letters that I wrote at this time to keep my friends and my family informed of my journey:

> I woke up in the middle of the night about 3:15 a.m. and lay in the bed, listening to the Houston night noises. I heard a train whistle blow as the lonesome, early morning engine left town. I thought, "How nice it would be to jump on that train and to go far, far away—away from MD Anderson and my Cancer, away so that my poor body could

heal from the devastations of this awful disease, and away from the pain, the needles, the blood, the fevers, and the sickness that comes with all Cancers". However, I know that with the return of the light of day, I will get up and will eat my All-Bran Cereal and go to MD Anderson for another chemo treatment in the real world. I know that I can only dream of this nightmare ending right now. This time in my life is not fun, and I hate to go through it, but I know that I must do it so that I will never have Cancer again. I am better off than most of the people that I see at MD Anderson. I will be well again in the summer. I believe that I will be cured of Cancer. A lot of the people at MD Anderson fight Cancer over and over again. I am amazed and impressed with their strength and love of life. Just being at MD Anderson around all of these Cancer patients is a learning experience that affects me profoundly.

I have made my "mark off" chart, and I have ten lines of squares to mark off. This chart is a day chart, so I can mark off another square each morning. I nearly have the first line finished. When I get all of the squares x'd off, I will be finished with my chemotherapy. Next week, my doctor says that I will lose my hair. What am I going to look like with a bald head? What will I do?

Side Effects Already

At this stage of the chemo game, I lost the feeling in the end of my right index finger. This wasn't too bad, but I never realized before how much I used that finger. I had played the piano for many years, and although I didn't have one in our apartment, I hoped that the neuropathy in my finger would not affect my playing. Peripheral neuropathy is a condition that causes tingling, burning, weakness, or numbness in the hands and/or the feet. It is a known side effect with the taxane drugs like Taxol. My chemotherapy book that I referenced often reported that these conditions would sometimes lessen over time and may be temporary. I hoped that mine would be temporary. My index finger actually hurt when I used it. It is an important finger—it is the one that I used on the TV clicker. Ha ha. This finger was only the first of several appendages that lost feeling as the chemo progressed.

There were days when I was sick (just did not feel good and ran a little fever). On Wednesday of that week, we were scheduled to go out to dinner with Paul's friends, Dick and Mary Frances. I nearly stayed home because I just did not feel good, but I hated to ruin Paul's planned evening with his old college friends. I went even though I didn't feel up to it and amazingly began to feel better at the restaurant with our friends. I always got so bored when I didn't feel good. At these times, I couldn't do anything but sit around, and that surely was no fun at all.

As it turned out, Dick and Mary Francis became good friends of mine, and we enjoyed their company many times while we were in Houston. Mary Frances worked as a project manager at MD Anderson and loved the place. It is so sad that a few years later, she died from lung Cancer that metastasized to her brain. I am glad that I didn't have a crystal ball that would have shown me her future. I don't think that I could have handled knowing that my friend was soon to die from Cancer, the very disease that I was fighting.

I continued to meet each week with my counselor and to explore my feelings and fears about Cancer and its effect on me. At this time, just like my doctor had said, I began to lose my hair. Hair began to fall from my head faster than the leaves fall from the beautiful trees in the fall. It was falling out by the handfuls. When I made the bed on that Friday morning, about two and a half weeks after I had taken my first chemo treatment, I was startled to find that the place where I lay my head looked like a shaggy old dog's bed with hair everywhere. When I washed my hair that morning, my fingers were entangled in masses of hair that just fell out. I had gone by the MD Anderson Beauty Shop the day before and had had my hair cut really short. It looked really cute, but as I continued to lose more hair each day, I knew that it wasn't going to be cute very long.

While I was at the beauty shop, I had attended a scarf-tying and head-covering class. I also had tried on wigs, but I just couldn't bring myself to get one while I still had hair. I realized that morning that I would have to get one soon.

The next morning, I awoke to find that my bed covers were piled up with hair. I had to dust the hair off so that I didn't get it in my nose and my mouth. I could hardly believe that I had any hair left at all on my head, but I had about a hundred hairs still hanging on. I shrugged and said to myself, "Oh, well. *I have never heard of anyone not growing their hair back*, so I am going to assume that my hair will grow back someday also. I may look funny, *but it will be okay again sometime.*"

MD Anderson was very good in offering many, many free services to its patients. When I had hair, I went to the beauty shop in the basement of the hospital and got my hair cut for free. They would also give me a wig when I wanted it. They offered training on ways to make yourself attractive when you were bald. If you fight Cancer, take advantage of all of these "help" programs. Fighting Cancer is very hard. You need help and advice. *Don't ever be too proud to accept caring people's support.*

I also began to suffer from itching. As a result, my arms and legs became scratched. My face had red blotches on it that I hated, but I assumed that all of this was just "fun with chemo." I had diarrhea again and felt poorly on Tuesday and Thursday. I had suffered from a headache on Wednesday afternoon. I thought that by Saturday, the chemo medicines from Monday would nearly all be out of my body. I began to feel better at the end of each week. At this time, Saturday and Sunday were my best days of the week. And each Monday, I had to go back to the hospital for another four—to five-hour chemo treatment. Yuck!

A Rude Awakening—The Bill

I received an itemized bill from MD Anderson that contained the costs of my first chemo treatment. I was shocked to find out that the bag of Taxol alone cost nearly $3,000.00. With each treatment, I was given lots of medicines to help counteract the bad side effects of the Taxol, and of course, there were also administration costs. From this bill, each weekly chemo treatment would cost about $4,000. The last statement that we had gotten from my insurance company showed bills from MD Anderson totaling $19,940.25. This statement covered parts of my mastectomy. We regularly got these insurance reports several times a week, but I had really not paid too much attention to them before. I didn't have any idea what this illness had cost, but it had been very expensive. Thank God that I had insurance.

I had gone all of my working life and had really not ever used my health insurance. I was always healthy. However, in 2003 and 2004, I used my health insurance. Having this good insurance (an 80/20 plan that didn't exclude anything) left my mind free to fight. I didn't have to worry about how we were ever going to pay for my treatments. I don't know what people did who didn't have medical insurance. Not having insurance would have made things VERY HARD for me.

We had just about finished paying off the doctors and the hospital in Durango for the Cancer treatments that I had back there before we got this particular bill from MD Anderson. Figuring out these insurance payments and bills was very, very complicated. I thought that a CPA would have had a hard time matching insurance payments to bills, etc. It was too complex for my chemo-affected brain. I didn't really want to spend my "up" time working through doctors, hospitals, and lab bills.

So far, our insurance company had been very good. We had fairly large deductibles that we had to pay and, of course, co-pays, but the bills had not yet been too much of a burden. My company-paid insurance co-payment (as a retiree) would go up dramatically for me the next year in 2004, but I was thankful that I would at least still have insurance. I had worked for forty years and never really used my health insurance. I guessed that I was finally catching up on all of those premiums that I had paid. It doesn't take long to catch up when one has Cancer.

My Marriage Anniversary and "Normal" Life

Saturday, November 15, was Paul and my seventeenth wedding anniversary, and we celebrated by going to see the movie *Master and Commander*, starring Russell Crowe, in the afternoon. Paul loved this movie since he used to race sailboats competitively. Nothing is more pleasurable to him than the sight of a fast ship breasting high seas with the low deck spraying water behind. Our anniversary celebration was simple and quiet. That evening Paul prepared dinner that we shared, just the two of us. We didn't have a lot of energy to spend in celebrating our 17 years of marriage. All of our energies were spent battling my Cancer.

BREAST CANCER: THE UNPLANNED JOURNEY - LESSONS LEARNED

Paul and I were getting accustomed to living in an apartment. We were comfortable in our little home. We were actually beginning to feel like the continual sounds of our neighbors above—walking, showering, and flushing their toilet—were a normal part of our lives. We even were aware of their intimacies and were no longer embarrassed. Being able to hear the lives of others and their personal interactions seemed really strange to us at first, but now it seemed "normal." We never met or even saw the people upstairs and next door, but we knew of their activities—and I guess that they knew of ours. We were truly "apartment dwellers" at that time.

I remained always thankful for all of the prayers, support through cards, e-mails and phone calls, and for the love that I received from my friends and family. I never felt alone in my battle. I got discouraged and I got tired, but I always knew that other people were pulling for me just as hard as they could. Knowing that I had support helped me. Paul, my husband, was fantastic. He continued to carry the main load of our business affairs and of my care. He did nearly all of the cooking and the cleaning. He was my constant companion and caretaker. I would go off by myself some, but he always worried about me while I was out of his sight. He was a very loving and sweet man, and he made my journey down this awful road easier.

My physical appearance got sicklier each day. I hated the red blotches that had appeared on my face, although I refused to let any of them ruin my smile. I smiled right through the red blotches. *My smile was my shield against Cancer.* Thank goodness that I had really good makeup so that I could do an expert job at covering things up when I went out. My hair at this time was getting very thin and scraggly, but I was determined *not* to hide alone in my apartment. I wanted to go on with life and the exciting things of the world did not happen inside my small Houston home. I hoped that people didn't notice my appearance and would not think badly of me or my illness.

MD Anderson has a wellness center, whose programs are free to Cancer patients. It was a wonderful place. At this time, I attended another journaling class and did another little writing this time on my "comfort bag." Everyone in the class was quite amused by my idea of this bag and its wonderful contents. This class was good for my spirits. I found that journaling was a way for me to express my feelings. As you know, I wrote prolifically during this time. I also participated in a Pilates class (an exercise/stretching class) at the Wellness Center. I wished that I could have attended this class every day.

I became very comfortable at MD Anderson. I began to learn to find my way through the maze of corridors and offices so that finding the pharmacy, the Breast Center, and the Transfusion Unit was easy. I even began to get acquainted with the receptionists and nurses. I also began to get acquainted with the patients there. And even though they didn't openly talk, when you were able to get them to talk, everyone was really friendly. All the people there had Cancer, and we had a lot of "in common" experiences. I was never embarrassed about looking sick or tired at MD Anderson. There were lots of people there just like me, and everyone understood about the "Cancer condition."

The specter of death was never very far away in the world of Cancer at MD Anderson. You couldn't talk to very many people on any given day before you ran into someone who was dying. I was amazed that everyone remained so strong amidst all of this strife and trouble. Learning to face death from Cancer is a fact of life for people at MD Anderson. I think that I have even become accustomed to this dark air that hangs there continuously. This darkness and fear makes everyone aware that life is fragile and must be appreciated. People who have Cancer have different values than busy people out in the working world. *People with Cancer enjoy the simple things—a short, sweet conversation, a child's smile, a lovely flower, and a hug.* Living in the world of Cancer, the world at MD Anderson, has affected me in many positive ways.

My Fourth Chemo Treatment

Bad Weather

Monday, November 17, Houston was assaulted with tornadic winds and down-pouring rains. Floods covered all the low-lying roads. The bayous raged and filled their banks to near overflowing. Traffic filled the streets and freeways so that soon, Houston traffic became a nightmare. Fortunately, Paul and I were at MD Anderson all day, so we missed the complications of this fall storm. Early that rainy morning, he dropped me at the hospital for my usual blood test and for my doctor's appointment. He then parked the car and walked in. We were inside the hospital the whole day.

Underarm Drainage

I also had to have my right underarm drained again. Before we left Houston for any reason, I always wanted to have everything with my health in as good a shape as I could get it, which always included draining the fluids from the right side underarm area. We were returning to Grapevine that week after my treatment, and I didn't want to have to go to the Grapevine Baylor Hospital with another Cancer emergency like I had earlier with my high fever episode and my "busted" boob. That Monday, the nurse drained nearly 250 cc of fluid from under my right arm. In the previous drainings, the nurse had not been able to get all of the fluid to bleed out, but today everything broke loose and drained completely. I nearly had a flat underarm on the right side again.

Healing Hands

The next thing that I did on that Monday chemo day was to go to the Wellness Center and to receive a "Healing Hands" session. I had never participated in this kind of treatment before. I had attended a luncheon training session on this technique, which entitled me to a treatment session. I was met in one of the quiet rooms in the Wellness Center by a small Hawaiian-looking lady named Noyme Smith. Obviously, her husband wasn't Hawaiian. She had a table for me to lie on that raised me up to her waist level. She instructed me to take off my shoes, and she took off hers also. She told me to lie down on the table and my only job was to "relax" completely. She turned the lights down, turned on some soothing sounds (of water running, I think), and went to work.

I shut my eyes and tried to relax. She stood over me and moved her hands over my body in my energy field. I had my clothes on. She didn't touch me. She didn't make any sounds. She simply moved her hands in and out of my energy field. I could feel where her hands were over my body even though she wasn't touching me. She had asked me about what was wrong with my body. I told her that my right knee and my right elbow hurt and that I had suffered from a headache that prior week.

As we got into the treatment, I told her that I was losing my hair and that I had fluid drainage under my right arm. She worked on those special areas also. I lay on the table and felt her hands moving over all the parts of my body (even though she didn't touch me). When she got to my breast areas, of course, she could see that I had undergone a double mastectomy, and she spent a longer time working in that area. It actually felt like her hands were rubbing my muscles under the skin. It was all very soothing and very relaxing. I was completely dressed, but it was like I could feel her hands inside my skin. I always knew where she was even though I had my eyes shut.

As I lay on the table, I listened to the Houston storm rage outside. It thundered and rained hard enough that I could hear the water beating down on the roof. I heard many sirens blasting, so I knew that many ambulances were leaving this hospital center in response to storm accidents. I had seen on the news channel that a storm that contained tornadoes was moving into our Houston area. The storm did not distract Noyme, so I just lay and listened to it and was thankful for the relaxing and healing time that I was enjoying. Noyme finished her treatment by going completely around my body with her hands. I got up and left feeling much more relaxed but not changed. I had no idea what effect her treatment would have on me.

Actual Chemo Treatment

The next item on the agenda that day was my chemo treatment. When we got to my room, we watched the storm reporting on the TV. Chemo started as usual, with me requesting the IV Starter people (a special hospital team that put in IVs in difficult cases) to get an IV started in my arm. This time, they poked and poked. They stuck three different veins in my lower arm and did not get a satisfactory vein. Two of the veins they stuck had been used previously and could not be used again. Apparently, the Taxol scars the vein so that it cannot be used for chemo again. They finally ended up using a vein that was nearly under my left armpit. It was in a strange place, but it worked.

My treatment cocktail changed a little that week. I received two bags of Benadryl, the regular bag of Tagament, the bag of Decadron (the steroid), and the regular bag of Taxol. Because my veins were just about all used up and because of my reactions to Benadryl, the treatment lasted from 12:00 p.m. until nearly 6:00 p.m. When I was done that evening, it was dark and awful outside. The traffic was bumper to bumper. Many of the freeways in Houston were closed because of high water. It had rained over eight inches while I was in the hospital. Fortunately, we didn't have to drive but one mile to get to our home. We did not have to get on a freeway. It took us quite a while to drive just that one mile, but we got home uneventfully, and we were thankful.

Our apartment was fine. There was no wind or rain damage. The bayou beside our apartment complex was full and raging, but it did not leave its banks. I had never seen it full like this before. Weeds and grass grew along the sides of the bayou above the cement sides. The water was covering all of the grass. The traffic on the freeways was stopped from wrecks and floodwaters. The reporters told everyone that the normal hour commute from work had become a four—to five-hour commute. We were thankful to get home that night and into our covered parking and our small apartment out of harm's way.

Best Week Ever

This week turned out to be the best week that I had experienced since I started the chemo treatments. Usually I went home after a treatment, ate a little supper, and then went to bed for the night. However, that Monday evening I stayed up until ten, working to get things packed so that we could leave the next morning. I had energy and I felt good. I had diarrhea, but I didn't feel sick. This good feeling continued all week. We drove to Grapevine very early Tuesday morning (the day after my fourth chemo treatment), and I stayed awake with Paul the whole way. I cleaned our Grapevine house, walked, and visited almost normally with our old friends in Grapevine. I was very, very happy.

I felt almost well again. I had no sore knees or joints, no headaches or backaches, no weakness or sickness. I took this good time as a special blessing. I had two "well/normal" days. I had my "before Cancer" levels of energy. I could work as I had before I started chemo. It was *wonderful*. I felt so very good. I couldn't believe it. I felt that I could do this chemo if I could keep getting a few of these days. I didn't have to spend a lot of the day in the bed. I felt good Thursday morning, but by Thursday afternoon, I was showing the old signs of a "chemo" body and had to cut Thursday evening short.

Friday morning, I woke up with a very sore right knee and right elbow. I had no energy and only walked because Marilyn, my friend, would not hurry and didn't seem to mind my slowness. But I did walk our usual distance! I went to bed for the afternoon. My bag of energy was gone completely. I wondered if the Healing Hands treatment that I had experienced had made the difference. I really should have explored getting more of these treatments, but I didn't. I didn't

BREAST CANCER: THE UNPLANNED JOURNEY - LESSONS LEARNED

know how much they cost, and I didn't think that my insurance would have paid for them. However, getting them might have made chemo easier.

We remained in Grapevine for the rest of the week. I worked hard at seeing as many of my good friends as I could. I tried to see all of the area grandkids also, even though their lives were very busy.

The weather was marvelous—"Chamber of Commerce" weather. The nights were cold, and the days were sunny and brisk. The trees were yellow and the fallen leaves were blowing in the autumn wind. Paul's camellias had a few blooms on them in our courtyard. Life was good in Texas that week. We returned to Houston on Sunday, after we had attended our home church. I had really enjoyed the "vacation" from Houston and the unplanned journey.

My hair continued to fall out. I guessed that I must have had about a million or a billion hairs. I just couldn't believe that I was losing so much hair and still had any at all left on my head. I wore a hat to church. I was the only one there in a big congregation with a hat on my head. This nearly hairless situation really complicated my getting-ready process. To dress for church, it already took me an extra fifteen minutes in the "dressing" process to get my false boobs in place and looking right. Now I had to add an extra thirty minutes for me to create and put together headgear for my outfits. Hats and turbans and scarves can be really cute, but they must be "put together" and styled. I did get a little better at this as I went along, but right now, it was a major job for me to get dressed up to go out.

My "dress up" life was quite involved now, with false boobs and false hair coverings, and it kept me laughing on the outside because my other option was just to cry. *I now had the job of working to be "bald and beautiful"* like Sandy, the lady I had met when I first went to church in Durango in 2000. I really looked awful with my almost bald head, but I hoped and prayed that this condition would pass. I hoped that a new me would emerge at the end of the unplanned journey. I was comforted with the fact that at least in Houston, I was among the Cancer patients at MD Anderson most of the time, and they knew all about my conditions. They were not afraid or startled with it. I did not look out of place to have no hair at MD Anderson. I began to feel "at home" among the Cancer people.

Chapter 30

LET THE CHEMO KILL MY CANCER

Taxol Treatment Number Five

Central Line Catheter Reinsertion

Monday, November 24, I reported to MD Anderson at 8:00 a.m. I had an appointment to get my central line catheter installed a second time. You may remember that my central line catheter was removed in the Grapevine Baylor Hospital when I had the high fever infection episode the last of October. I had been getting my chemo treatments as IVs that they inserted in my arm each week. However, the veins in my arm were wearing out. I very much wanted the ease of having central line catheter again.

The first step in this process was for us to learn how to care for it. We had to receive another lovely review of the Philippine "strict nurse" routine, which showed us how to change the dressing, insert a daily "cleaning out shot," etc. Paul did not have to perform another change to prove that he could handle the job this time, thankfully. When he was asked about whether he needed training on this, he adamantly told everyone that he had already been qualified. He in no way wanted to go through any of their training again.

I watched with great interest as this little nurse very efficiently prepared me, the room, and herself for my surgery. It was a show in itself. Watching her gown and glove up without touching anything was really a spectacle to see. I stretched and held my head up to watch the complete performance while I lay on the surgical bed. She was good. I was quite confident that everything that went on under her supervision was completely sterile.

When I and the room were all prepared, the doctor came in and maybe stayed eight minutes. He deadened my shoulder area, stuck in the catheter, and left before I had time to think about it. It hurt a little but was nothing bad. The nurse stitched the catheter down and bandaged me. It was all done in about an hour. I then went down to x-ray to make sure that the line was in the vein correctly. They would not free me to go to chemo until after they had checked the x-ray. It was a busy morning, but I made it to chemo by eleven thirty.

Week Five Chemo Treatment

Week five of chemo went by without a snag. I didn't have to have an IV needle installed in my arm now because I had the central line catheter. This made my chemo time anywhere from twenty minutes to an hour shorter. I actually finished receiving the chemo that day a little after 4:00 p.m. I got the Decadron (the steroid) again. I had a small reaction to the Taxol in treatment four, when I suffered lower back pain during the infusion. They gave me Decadron to counteract it. Because I felt so good after receiving the steroid, my doctor decided that this should be a regular part of my treatment. However, the steroid causes weight gain, and I was concerned about that. I also took Tagament (for my stomach acid) in this treatment.

The treatment lasted from 12:00 p.m. to 4:15 p.m. I slept through the last hour and a half. Paul was there watching over me all of the time. Therefore, I was relaxed. Thanksgiving week went quietly. I could not get another "Healing Hands" treatment, because all of the qualified therapists were on vacation. I did do another counseling session, which continued to help me in unraveling and seeing through all the issues that I had experienced with this Cancer. My counselor was very helpful.

I did have a very good Tuesday and Wednesday again. I was not sick. I didn't have quite as much energy as I had enjoyed in the fourth week, but I did okay. On Friday, I worked getting Paul's bike completely repaired (I bought a new chain and installed it) and then rode it home from the bike shop. I ended up riding over five miles. It was a perfect day for bike riding. I rode on a bike trail that ran along the Braeswood Bayou, away from the Houston traffic.

Thanksgiving Day, 2003

We went to Sondra and Peter's (number 2 son's) house for Thanksgiving Day. We enjoyed a delicious lunch with them and their three boys, Fritz, Foster, and Grant. I brought homemade pumpkin pie and cranberry sauce. Sondra fixed turkey and dressing, yams, mashed potatoes, and green bean casserole. It was all very good. When we went around the table, saying what we were thankful for, Paul said that he was thankful that I had no more Cancer tumors in my body, and *I thanked God for all of my wonderful family, especially for my grandchildren, and for my friends who had helped me through hard times this year.* And you must note that I got through this little speech without crying. Paul and I watched a little of the cowboy game and then came home. I was tired again.

Sores and Lesions and Extreme Fatigue

On that Thanksgiving Day at Peter's house, when I was wearing a really pretty straw hat with a fancy band on it, my head got to itching and hurting. I took off my hat and felt of my scalp and suddenly felt bumps all over it. I had my new daughter, Sondra, check my head out for me, and she reported that I had sore-looking red bumps all over my scalp. Well, if that wasn't the pits! I had no hair and now my scalp was breaking out with ugly sores. Later that week, I also developed red splotches (sores) on my arms and a few even on my legs. These red places seemed to ulcerate from the inside out and just peel. Little white heads came up and broke and ran. What a mess! These new sores never bled or made real sores; they just ulcerated and peeled all of the time. Not only was I bald but now my scalp and my body were covered with red lesions. I suffered through this on Friday, Saturday, and Sunday.

All the time I wore soft scarves to cover the sores up, and I washed my hair with my special (easy on the skin and nonallergenic) face-skin wash from BeautiControl. It felt better after the washing, but the sores did not go away. I began to feel like the Old Testament character Job again. Was God allowing the Devil to test me just like Job had been tested? In this Bible story there is a verse about Job breaking out with running lesions and sores all over his body. This verse haunted me. I also knew that in the end, Job had been all right, but I knew too well his pain and suffering described in the Bible, and wanted no part of that. However, I didn't seem to have had any choice in the matter.

Saturday afternoon, I came home and took a nap and then went to bed for the night about eight thirty. I just had no energy. On Sunday, I got up and went to church but did not enjoy it. I was just too tired. We came home, and I went to bed for the afternoon. I got up only to eat supper and to watch a little TV. However, after supper, my neck froze up and got to hurting awfully. I took pain pills that only helped a little. I went to bed and took a sleeping pill in order to get to sleep. The strange pains that I got with Taxol were really surprising. I never knew where they would hit. The ones on my back and neck were severe enough that I could not endure them without strong pain pills. I looked forward to seeing my doctor again.

I went to see the doctor on Monday, December 1. My head had swollen ugly breakout bumps all over it. I also had similar sores on my arms and even a few on my legs. Apparently, I had a hair follicle infection. This affected everywhere that I had hair follicles. The lesions that I had developed on my arms and legs were caused by the same infection that had first infected the hair follicles on my bald head. These awful red spots were not normal and hopefully could be healed with medicine. The doctor gave me Tetracycline, an antibiotic to help this. He prescribed the old time pHisoHex wash also. I had trouble getting my prescription for pHisoHex filled because the drug store no longer carried it. They had to order it for me, and eventually I was able to get it.

Nearly all of the hair on my body—my pubic hair, my eye lashes, and the hair on my arms and legs—had fallen out. Lots of the places where I had once had hair were now covered with red, awful sores. I still had eyebrows, and I was thankful for that. A person really looks "chemo sick" when he does not have any facial hair.

I reported my two "absolutely no energy" days of Saturday and Sunday to my doctor. I began to understand why it is so hard for me to get anything done. I was not writing much at this time. I was not doing any sewing. I had no energy, and I didn't feel good most of the time. I just sat around and felt miserable. I was getting through my time, but I wasn't doing it well. When I had a day that was good, it was wonderful and I enjoyed it to the fullest. *The good days kept me going through the bad days*. I had been feeling so guilty from not getting things done. I decided after talking to the doctor that I was just too hard on myself. I had hardly ever spent a day in bed before, but now I was spending lots of afternoons and evenings there. Fortunately, Paul was completely loving and understanding about all of this. He never pushed me to do anything, but even he really enjoyed the days where I did have energy.

The doctor, in reaction to my complaint, ordered more blood tests. I was also getting a consult with the Physical Therapy Department to work out an exercise program for me during this chemo. They have a really nice gym and workout area here that I could use if I worked with a therapist. Hopefully all of this would help me.

MD Anderson had a "fatigue clinic," and they were currently doing a study which I qualified for. My doctor suggested that I might want to look into that, and I decided to do that. The study was studying the use of Ritalin as a stimulant during chemo treatments to help fatigue.

Sixth Chemo Treatment

Chemo Treatment and Life

I finally got around to taking my chemo treatment that sixth Monday, and everything went normally. I had completed two lines of my "mark off" chart. I could see my X's getting nearer to the end of my chemo timeline chart. By now, getting chemo treatments had settled into some kind of normal activity. I felt pretty good on Tuesdays and Wednesdays, but my energy went down after that. By Saturday and Sunday, I was "all done in." I managed to always go to church, but I just sat there and didn't kneel and stand with the congregation. Most afternoons were spent in bed napping. I got up for supper and maybe sat in my lounge chair for a little TV watching afterward. I didn't go into the grocery store anymore when Paul went. I sat in the car and waited. My right elbow and my right knee hurt a lot of the time.

Chemo had robbed me of all of my energy. My hair had pretty much all fallen out. It looked absolutely awful. However, I would live with this. I was experimenting with all kinds of hats and scarves. A friend had loaned me a wig, and I thought about buying another one. Paul didn't seem to be upset with me, but I hated to see my reflection in the mirror. Next summer, I hoped that this would all be over, and I thought that I might look back on this as a learning experience.

I couldn't imagine looking back on this time with any kind of joy or appreciation. Luckily, I had the foresight and optimism to hope that I might someday realize the good in this experience.

My Birthday

On December 4, I turned sixty-one years old. Paul and I spent a quiet day together. I made a few calls, received calls from my children, received several birthday cards, and opened a few gifts. It was a nice birthday. Having celebrations during this year of Cancer seemed a little strange to me. Celebrations just didn't seem to fit into my world of fatigue, falling out hair, and a failing body. My friends from my water aerobics class in Durango, the Mermaids, called and sang "Happy Birthday" to me. That was a real treat! Paul fixed steak for supper, and we watched TV that evening. I didn't even really feel like going out to see the Christmas tree lighting at Rice University. An excerpt from my letter from that time period follows:

> I have completed week six of my Taxol treatments. My body continues to change as it stores more and more of the Taxol. Chemotherapy drugs are basically poisons that attack and kill cells. They do, hopefully, attack and kill the Cancer cells. However, they also attack and kill a lot of other cells. They apparently work differently in every body. Since the doctors cannot find any other Cancer cells in my body now, they have no idea whether the chemotherapy drugs are doing what they are supposed to—killing hidden Cancer cells—but they can see that it is affecting other cells in my body.
>
> Very soon, doctors at MD Anderson will institute a new treatment that will require all Cancer patients to take chemotherapy before any surgery is performed. They want to determine before they cut out the Cancer, a chemo regime that works against each person's Cancer. This seems awfully smart to me. I just had my Cancer about six months too soon and did not get to MD Anderson soon enough to undergo this new treatment process. When they treat the Cancer with chemo before they take it out with surgery, they can determine which chemo cocktail is effective in reducing that particular Cancer. I certainly hope that my chemo cocktail is killing any Cancer cells that might have escaped into my body from my breast Cancer. I am going through this awful treatment to purchase insurance against my ever having breast Cancer again. Now you may ask how I could ever have breast Cancer again because I no longer have any breasts. But breast Cancer kills a person by metastasizing (or beginning to grow again) in some other part of the body. Breast Cancer can spread to the liver, to the lungs, to the brain, to the bones, or other places. It is breast Cancer (just like the original Cancer that grew first in the breast), but now it is growing in another place in my body. It has metastasized.

I must now describe myself since all of you fortunately can't see how I look. I have gone through the "losing my hair" stage. The hair on my head fell out in handfuls for about two weeks. It really made a mess. My hair got thinner and thinner until you could see my scalp everywhere. I have a few hairs left, but they are scattered, and there are only a few of them. My head is not smooth and clean like a bald man's head. My head has some hair all over it, just not enough to cover the scalp. I had never seen my round head without hair before. It was a shock to get accustomed to seeing myself with a bald head. I finally now can look at myself in the mirror, but it's not a pretty sight. I cut off the hair that was left so that it is all about one-half inch long all over my head. It is light in color and doesn't show much.

Head Sore Update and My Current Appearance

After taking all of the antibiotic and washing faithfully with the pHisoHex, the sores on my head and arms got better. They had not all gone away, however, so the doctor prescribed another round of the antibiotic. I decided that *this disease was the scourge of the Devil, if ever there was one*. I continued to have real sympathy for Job.

During week six of my chemo, I started waking up every morning with red, sunken eyes. It looked like I had been crying all of the time or had suffered a severe allergic reaction. I had seen these sunken red eyes on other chemo patients. I thought that this was just a normal reaction to chemo. But with all these other physical marks, I now really looked like a "Cancer" patient. Because of the sores on my scalp, I hadn't worn a wig yet. I wore lots of scarves and hats. I like hats and have quite a few that I had gathered over the years. Now I was really using my collection. Before now, the hats had just decorated my closet. I also wore hats for warmth these days. I never knew before that my hair provided so much heat to my head and body. My head was now cold a lot of the time. With red sunken eyes, no hair, and skin that was pale and blotchy, with small red peeling lesions everywhere, I now looked like I belonged at MD Anderson. I was tired most of the time. I could still smile, but I looked like a person who was deep into the fight against Cancer.

As I said above, taking chemo is like poisoning your body a little more each week. I wouldn't do it, except that I looked at chemo as my insurance against ever having breast Cancer again. When I made this statement in my breast Cancer support group meeting, everyone just gasped and said that I shouldn't say that I will never have breast Cancer again. My thoughts at the time were "Why am I going through this awful chemotherapy if it isn't buying me something? I want it to get rid of all the loose breast Cancer cells so that I never have breast Cancer again ". I prayed every day that God would use this chemo to kill all of the Cancer cells that existed anywhere in my body. I did not want to go on this unplanned journey again.

Life Continues On

Despite my being tired and my ugly appearance, life continued. My life was simple. I spent a lot of time sitting and sleeping. There were many days in which I did not stick my nose out of the apartment. On those days, it just felt good to sleep most of the day and to rest. *I thanked God for the ability to sleep.* Sleep allowed time to pass quickly and easily. I was peaceful in sleep. During this time, I thought that if I could be Rip Van Winkle and just sleep through this entire experience, I would. I was sleeping a lot now and that was a blessing.

I continued to ride my bike on the days when I could. The weather in Houston was nearly perfect that winter. We had cool nights and warm days. I began physical therapy treatments to improve the flexibility in my arms and to try and to fight the fatigue. I had never experienced therapy before. It was a learning experience for me. The following is an excerpt of personal thoughts from my newsletter at this time:

> I am very lucky. Paul is an excellent caregiver and continues down this Cancer road right beside me. He is patient beyond all expectations. Our life right now is *not* exciting or fun. A good day for us consists of me doing just a couple of things and of my feeling fairly well. We go to MD Anderson regularly. We see a few movies. And so far, we have managed to get to church each Sunday, although that gets harder and harder for me as I get deeper into the chemo. My energy level seems to be the lowest on Sundays. Seeing our family and a few friends is really a treat for us. Paul never fusses or complains about our boring, boring life right now. Thank God for Paul.

> I am working to get out my Christmas cards. I have so many people whom I want to say thank you to for their support of me during this year that sending out cards this year is a big job. However, I have lots of time right now. I left my traditional Christmas card list in Grapevine. I plan on sending cards to my Cancer supporters this year. We received our first Christmas card this week. We haven't gotten a tree yet, but I do plan on putting up something for Christmas. My counselor advises me that I should find something to put on my tree or in my Christmas decorations that will always be a symbol of this Cancer year. I think that this is a good idea. I should never forget this Cancer year of 2003, but for the life of me, cannot think what I want to add. How do I want to remember this Cancer Christmas of 2003?

> Life continues on. Children grow, new babies are born, and old people die. Each of us struggles in his own way to keep life vibrant and good. I struggle now against the last of the vestiges of the Cancer monster that invaded my body. *My battle takes time*

and must be fought one day at a time. And that is the way I am living my life. In my time chart, I am a little over one-fourth of the way done with my chemo. Time seems to crawl by for me.

I am finding it harder and harder to sit down at the computer to write. I am not good at answering my e-mails, although I do read and enjoy them all. My newsletters get shorter and farther apart.

Chapter 31

THE END OF A BAD YEAR

Treatment Number Seven

I took treatment number seven this last Monday, December 8. The doctor did not give me the steroid, Decadron. I took the Taxol without infusion symptoms. The Decadron in the past had given me a spurt of energy on Tuesday and Wednesday. I couldn't sleep easily or long on those nights, however. But then when the energy left, the symptoms from the Taxol were severe. And Friday, Saturday, and Sunday were really hard days for me.

Treatment Number Eight

Treatment number eight occurred as scheduled on December 15. At this point, I had only four more weeks of Taxol to go. I was tired most of the time. I was bald but at least my sores were getting better. I still had red spots on my face, arms, and legs, and I still had sunken, swollen, red eyes. I began to have numb toes, numb thumbs, and numb index fingers on my hands. I had very little energy and didn't do too much. One of the hard things for me to do was to look at myself in the mirror. I just could hardly stand to see the way I looked. I never thought that I could look so ugly. Thank goodness, Paul never seemed to notice it. He still lovingly called me his pet names of "Sweet B" and "Sunshine", even though my step had lost its lilt and I had no brightness about me now. In ways, I was glad that I was far away from my friends and family. I hoped that maybe by the time they saw me again, I would be over this terrible time in my life and would look a little more like I used to look.

I wrote about my baldness in one of my letters as follows:

> Chemo is *no* fun, but I am okay. I will make it through this treatment. I have lots of hats now. Thanks to all of you who have contributed to my stock. I have some especially warm hats that I wear even inside buildings. I get cold from not having hair on my head. *Please remember that a bad hair day is better anytime than a no-hair day.*

I now began my participation in a study to determine if Ritalin would help the joint pain and fatigue that accompanies chemo. It did seem to help me a little. At least that Sunday I had not stayed in bed the whole day like I had the Sunday before that when I had lain in my bed nearly all day. It was a good thing for me to have the strength to stay up on the weekends. The days before I had each chemo treatment seemed to be the hardest days for me.

Christmas at MD Anderson and At Our Apartment

Christmas was coming to Houston, and sometimes it was even cold. Christmas at MD Anderson was interesting. Remember that even during this bright and wonderful Christmas season, you still had all these very sick Cancer patients everywhere. You still had people with IV poles, robes, and house shoes where ever you looked. There were lots of people who wore hats and wigs because they had no hair. But at this time of year, among all of this pain and suffering at MD Anderson, you now saw Christmas trees, poinsettias, bright lights, and multicolored balls.

The hospital held a decorating contest between the different departments. The Physical Therapy Department had designed their own holiday Monopoly game and had decorated their waiting area with Monopoly money, houses, hotels, dice, and deeds. They renamed all the properties so that they were parts of MD Anderson. It was really cute. I didn't see all of the departments, but I was very impressed with the Physical Therapy Department's creative job in decorating for Christmas. They actually won the contest and were awarded a pizza party for everyone in the department.

The hospital lobby at MD Anderson included a high open atrium, and the staff had put a twelve-foot-tall Christmas tree there. They always had a lovely Yamaha Grand Piano in this bright area. At Christmas, the volunteer coordinator who manages the piano programming lined up over one hundred performers to come and play during the two weeks before Christmas. From about 11:00 a.m. until after 3:00 p.m., people came to play and sing. The performances that I saw were spectacular. I saw a trombone sextet; an acoustical guitar and flute ensemble; a tuba, bass, and trombone ensemble; a Madrigal group of singers in full costume singing a cappella; a male tenor with piano accompaniment; a violin player; a sixth-grade string band and choir; and numerous individual piano players.

I looked forward every time that I went to the hospital to taking a little time off and listening in this lovely open hall and enjoying the very entertaining and uplifting Christmas music. Being retired and doing absolutely nothing but Cancer, I had the time to enjoy some of these wonderful performances. These performers came and "played their drum" for the Cancer patients at MD Anderson just like the little boy came to play for baby Jesus in the song, "The Little Drummer Boy". These programs gave me a magnificent Christmas present. This was a very different Christmas, but it was enjoyable. It was a Christmas in the land of Cancer at MD Anderson.

I only put a few decorations up in our apartment. My traditional Christmas decorations were in Grapevine. We bought a small tree and a real pine wreath that were the centerpieces of our Christmas decorations. I had a small gathering of lovely long pink balls that I had tied together that hung on our front door. I wanted these pink balls to be my Cancer Christmas decoration to be hung year after year. Pink is never my "Christmas color" so these hanging balls will always be different—just like the Christmas of 2003 (my Cancer Christmas) will always be different from my normal Christmas celebrations. My experiences that year were something I would never forget. I got my Christmas cards finished and mailed. I somehow managed to finish a little Christmas shopping. Despite Cancer and the awful way that I felt and looked, Christmas was coming. This would not be a banner year at our house, but I would make it through.

Stolen Bikes

At this happy time of year, I went out to get on my bike one morning, and it was gone. My bicycle was stolen while it was chain locked to the bike rack in our apartment garage behind locked gates. The chain we had used was not big and heavy, but it was a metal chain. Later that week, Paul's bike was also stolen. I was very upset about being robbed. Recently, there had been two apartments in our complex that were broken into and two cars were vandalized in our parking lot. I had trouble believing that Houston was such an unsafe place. I felt absolutely safe and protected at MD Anderson, but I knew that I had to remember that when I stepped outside, I had better watch out. I learned that you have to always lock up everything. I am very thankful that we could afford to replace our bicycles. I hope that whoever took them really needed them. They were good bikes.

We went to a family Christmas celebration here with our Houston sons and their families on Saturday afternoon, December 20. We gathered at Sondra and Peter's house and shared a meal and gave presents to the children. I enjoyed it very much.

Treatment Number Nine

On Monday, December 22, I went to the hospital to receive my ninth infusion of chemo. The ravages of Taxol on my body continued. I constantly prayed at this time that Taxol would search my body and would kill any and all Cancer cells that might exist and that it would not harm any of my organs or the good tissue of my body. My fatigue seemed to be a permanent part of life. I didn't do a lot, and I tried not to worry about all of the "undone" things in our apartment. I now went to bed immediately after an early supper each day. I just felt better lying down. My eyes were still sunken and red. I could not wear eye makeup because if I tried to cover my awful eyes, they would mat up solid over the night. I had to soak them with water to open them the next morning. I suffered from some vomiting. The red splotches on my arms and face and legs remained. The sores on my scalp, however, had finally healed.

Christmas In Grapevine

We left Houston on Tuesday morning, December 23, and drove to Grapevine. It was winter there. It really felt cold to me when we arrived. We turned the heater up and got out our coats. I cuddled under lots of blankets when I got into my bed at night. The trees in Grapevine were bare and stark and gray. The knurled branches of the bare oak trees formed interesting figures in the cold winter sky. Our yard was filled with dried leaves that blew around, making the wind visible. Paul's magnificent camellia bushes were in full bloom and made our otherwise dead yard bright with natural Christmas color. The now old huge camellia bushes are usually covered with beautiful flowers in the middle of the winter. If the freezes are not too hard, the camellia buds form and develop perfectly and offer their fuchsia and light pink waxy multipetaled flowers at the least expected time of year. They were beautiful for me that year, and I cut some to take back to Houston to give to friends at MD Anderson. The flowers last in a small arrangement a long time.

When we left in October, the gardenias were blooming a second time that year. Our yard, a result of Paul's planning, planting, and work, certainly tried to add beauty to my life that hard, cold winter. We saw our family and visited with good friends. We ate Christmas dinner with John's (number five son) wife's family, the Daboubs, and had a wonderful time. John hosted our family Christmas on Saturday, December 27, at his home. He served prime rib to twelve adults and eight children. It was a delicious meal and was handled very gracefully. It was really nice to see my grown children being able to handle events as nicely or maybe even a little better than I could. Family traditions would continue after I was too old to handle them.

We somehow got through Christmas. This Christmas had not been a "Christmas card" time (with snow, mistletoe, and the family gathered around a bright tree). 2003 was the year of Cancer in my life, and it was finally about to end. I would continue the chemo to ensure that I never had Cancer again.

A Time of Contemplation

Because I rested a lot, I had time to think. I talked about Christmas 2003, its events, and my reactions to the things that happened in my newsletter that I wrote when we got back to Houston the last week of December. I would like to quote directly from these writings in the following:

> I could be sad and cry because of the many things that I cannot do or that have happened to me this year, but I choose to be as happy as I can and to enjoy the blessings that come my way instead. In talking to my newly converted Catholic son, John (number five son), I understand that suffering is a part of God's plan and that he uses suffering to teach us and to bring us to better places in life. John is my son who had trouble accepting that his mother had Cancer. John has to learn how to handle my tears. It is interesting that when John went to Midnight Christmas Mass this year, the priest talked about people who shed a lot of tears as being people who felt things deeply. John, of course, thought of me. I hope that it makes him more understanding of my watery eyes because I do think that maybe I feel things more deeply than some people. Anyway, I know that I am learning things from this time of suffering with my Cancer. I know that God has a plan for me through this. And I know that *I am learning patience and quietness.*
>
> It has been nice visiting with our old friends during this holiday season. One of them asked me some very pertinent questions that I want to answer. She asked, (1) "Are you mad at God for causing these awful things to happen to you?" She immediately followed this first question with another. (2) "I have known lots of other people that have had Cancer, but none of them have had so many bad things happen to them. If you weren't going to MD Anderson, I would think that your medical care had been bad. Why have all of these terrible things happened to you with this Cancer?" My friend then asked, (3) "How do you keep yourself 'up'? Don't you get awfully discouraged and blue and down when you are so sick for so long without any real hope of being better in the near future?"
>
> All of her questions were thrown out one after the other amid a busy group conversation, and fortunately, no one waited to hear my answers to them. The conversation turned to another topic quickly, and I wasn't looked upon to give answers. Quietness is something that I think that I am learning with this Cancer, and it was easy for me to sit and to listen to the ongoing, flowing conversation that immediately filled the table while I sat quietly and thought about my answers to her questions. I thought that these questions were important and are probably ones that

everyone has asked silently. Therefore, I felt the need to try and to answer them. These questions are certainly things that I have thought about and have lived with every day.

Question 1.

"Has this suffering affected your faith? Are you mad at God for causing these awful things to happen to you?"

My Answer

No, I am not mad at God for allowing this to happen to me. I believe that God puts us down here on earth and allows the natural laws of the earth to generally rule our lives. If we drink poison, we probably will die. If we run out in front of a car, we will be badly hurt or killed according to the natural laws. If Cancer gets in your body, if you take hormones that feed it, and if you do not find it, it grows and spreads through your body according to the natural laws of the earth. It wasn't necessarily God's will or plan that I got Cancer. It wasn't necessarily God's plan that the Cancer got so big and went out of my breasts into my lymph system. My Cancer happened under the natural laws of the earth. God didn't "give" me this Cancer.

Now I do believe that God has the power to intervene and to change the natural laws on earth. I do believe in *miracles*. However, I believe that they are special and don't happen every day. However, being at MD Anderson, where death is always just around the corner, where Cancer is the monster that is the opponent of every person here, and where God's intervention into the natural laws of earth occurs more frequently, I have become *very aware* that God performs miracles by using the superhuman skills and brains of doctors, nurses, and researchers. I also *know* that God gives some Cancer patients superhuman strengths of survival and healing. I *believe* that God and my surgeons were able to rid my body of all breast Cancer cells sometime between July 20, when I had my second lumpectomy that did not get all of the Cancerous tumor from my breast, and September 15, when I had my double mastectomy and lymph-node removals. I know that somehow, the Cancer tumors went away. All of the tissue that they took from my body during the double mastectomy and lymph-node removals revealed *no* Cancer cells or tumors. This was my *miracle*. Where had the Cancer that was obviously in my breast after the July 20 lumpectomy gone? The only thing that happened to me during this time medically was the hematoma that caused my breast to "bust" and was then followed by the cleaning out of this infection.

Maybe in taking out the infected cells in my breast on August 14, my surgeon also took out the last remaining Cancer cells. I don't know. Maybe God just reached down and killed all of the Cancer cells that were left. I believe the pathology lab reports that I received from Durango (which said that there still might be Cancer cells in my breasts because the surgeon did not get clear margins). MD Anderson checked and rechecked these early findings and found no discrepancies. Maybe between July 20 and September 15, God killed all of the remaining Cancer cells in my breasts and lymph nodes. I do not know. How else does one explain that there were no more parts of Cancer tumors in the breast area of my body on September 15?

I do not blame God for my Cancer. I will remain close to Him during this unplanned journey. I will not allow Cancer to separate me from my God. The Cancer has affected my faith but not in a negative way. I am lucky enough to have probably had a miracle occur in my life.

Question 2.

"I have known lots of other people that have had Cancer, but none of them have had so many bad things happen to them. If you weren't going to MD Anderson, I would think that your medical care had been bad. Why have all of these terrible things happened to you with this Cancer?"

My Answer

As my life and battle of actually fighting the Cancer slows down in this chemo stage, this particular question weighs on my mind some. I don't really know for sure what the answer is, but I will relate the answers that I have come up with at this moment. I do not think that I have had bad doctors or bad care in my Cancer experience either in Durango or here at MD Anderson. Take first the incident where my right breast burst. This is an unusual happening! I do think that the doctor in Colorado might have released me before he was sure that my swelling right breast was going to go down. I know that the last time that I saw him, I thought that my right breast was too enlarged and gorged from the second lumpectomy, but he did not seem concerned and assured me that in time, it would go down. If I had been in Colorado, I would have insisted that he look at it again before it ruptured. However, being in Grapevine, eight hundred miles from him, seeing him was not an option. I had called him about three the afternoon before the evening that it burst. When he called back about eight that evening and talked to Paul, he advised Paul to get me into see a doctor "sooner rather than later." Of course, by then, I was already attending my meeting in Dallas, and

Paul didn't have a way to easily reach me. A hematoma occurs randomly and is not necessarily the fault of the surgeon or the hospital (according to my doctor daughter). I don't know why I had the infection in this second lumpectomy site, but I did. The hematoma might have occurred because after the first lumpectomy, I discovered that I was allergic to tape. After the second lumpectomy, the nurses bandaged my breast without the very tight tape bandage that they had used the first time. This looser bandage after the surgery might have caused the extra internal bleeding and the hematoma. Who knows? The care I received after the breast burst was good at the ER in Grapevine, Texas. I reported to MD Anderson as soon as I could, the following Thursday, and the surgeon there immediately scheduled me for surgery that evening. I couldn't have had better care than that. Even though the care after the surgery was a bit bizarre, we had to take out and re-stuff five yards or whatever amount it took to fill the hole of gauze/tape into the open breast each day; the procedure worked. I got rid of the infection, and the hole healed from the inside out. It was still open when I went in on September 15 to have the double mastectomy.

My surgery for the double mastectomy went very normally except for my wake-up hallucinations. These could have been a manifestation of the awful fears that I had before the surgery. Unfortunately, I did not talk about these fears to anyone. I was very scared that I would die during or immediately after this surgery. Only my daughter, Mary Joy, and two of my other friends, Mary Lee Hamisch and Cathey Daboub, had any inkling of these fears. I worked frantically before the surgery to get my life in order, to get everything done, and to be sure that I visited with all my family and friends. I do think my hidden but very real fears might have manifested themselves in these waking-up nightmare scenes that played in my mind and literally "scared me to death."

The infection that I got around the drains under my left arm five days after my mastectomy seemed minor because we caught it in the early stages. Somehow, from MD Anderson hospital, I picked up these bad germs. This slight infection was the first sign of the serious infection that would hit me later. This first outbreak, which occurred while we were still in Houston, sent me to the ER at MD Anderson. My experience at the Houston MD Anderson ER was good, and I left the hospital that evening after seeing one of my own surgeons with a prescription for a ten-day supply of a powerful antibiotic, Augmentin, 825 mg. My surgical healing seemed normal until the antibiotic ran out. Exactly one day after the antibiotic was completed, all of a sudden, I started running the high fever that reached 103.8 before the ER got it turned around. This attack hit in a matter of minutes. I felt fine, and then I got chilled and started physically shaking. After a couple of frantic calls, Paul took me to the ER here in Grapevine. You know the story from there. I spent five days in the hospital and was diagnosed to have a negative-rod Staph infection. I picked up this infection sometime in my stay at MD Anderson with the mastectomy surgery. It lay dormant, just quietly building up its strength while I took the Augmentin. When the antibiotic was gone from my system, the bad infection took off like gangbusters. That is the reason that I had such high fever with the "out of the clear" attack. I think that the sores (the hair follicle infection) that I got was just a side effect of the chemotherapy and a weakness in my body. My body has been ravaged over the past six months and is not in a strong position to fight off any infections or diseases.

The only answer that I can think of to this question of why I had so much trouble is that maybe God wants me to experience this one Cancer to the absolute fullest. In other words, maybe I am supposed to have all possible experiences with this one Cancer since I do not plan on having Cancer again. Maybe all of these different experiences will make my book richer and more complete. Maybe I am just a good storyteller, and everyone knows about all of my hardships. With other people, you probably don't hear about all of the problems that happen. I am so open and communicative that the world knows about all of my experiences. I know that my answers to why will probably change with time. I suspect that I will ask and answer these same questions many times in the future. These are real questions in my life.

Question 3.

"How do you keep yourself 'up'? Don't you get awfully discouraged and blue and down when you are so sick for so long without any real hope of being better in the near future?"

My Answer

The answer to this one is not too complicated. I get discouraged. When I hurt and do not feel good, I am more likely to find myself in the "dumper." Paul just hates it when I get down and cry, but I do it at times. I try to keep these times very private, and only Paul sees them. I try to stay happy and "up." When one walks the Cancer road at MD Anderson, fellow travelers that you meet buoy you up. There are so many people at this Cancer center with many worse situations than mine who demonstrate courage and an upbeat attitude. Their courage in the midst of such great trouble and travail and pain causes me to be obligated to stay up and positive with my simple Cancer, which I will survive. I can't cry about my little problems when they have so many more severe problems. My faith in God also helps me. I *know* that God will not give me more than

I am able to bear. I *know* this truth in my soul, but believe me, there are times when I could doubt if I let myself. It hurts Paul badly, however, when I get down, and I try not to do it any more than I just have to. My counseling sessions are a good place for me to cry and to unburden my soul in a safe place. My counselor doesn't get upset and isn't hurt from my honest tears and frustrations and cries of hurt. I have also made me a day chart of the time of all of my chemo treatments. It shows me a set number of days that I must endure before the chemo will end, and I will begin to get better. Being able to mark off the days on this chart is a help to keep me going. I know that there is an end somewhere down the line.

This has not been the greatest of Christmases, but it had its own teachings. Paul and I are lucky to have so many friends supporting me during this Cancer battle. My chemo time and miseries will pass. Very fortunately 2003 is just about over, and 2004 is bound to be a better year.

Chapter 32

HALFWAY DONE

The New Year, 2004

2003 had ended. Paul and I celebrated New Year's Day quietly in our apartment. We dined on black-eyed peas and homemade sweet yellow cornbread for lunch. Because I am a real Southerner, these are specialty dishes that are really good in my kitchen. I had enough energy that day to make our special lunch.

One of my resolutions for the New Year was to try to walk every day even when I didn't feel like it. The only time of the day when I had any energy at all was when I first got up in the morning. That was the time that I had to plan my walks. Even if I only walked a short way slowly, I thought that it would surely help me. It was a challenge to walk on Friday, January 2, because my right knee hurt. However, I walked anyway, and after I finished the walk, my knee actually felt better. I hoped that I would be able to keep this resolution. If we did not have other morning obligations like doctor's appointments or church or garage selling, I planned for us to go walking. Paul and I both badly needed the exercise.

Treatment Number 11

On January 5, 2004, on schedule, I took treatment eleven of Taxol! Hooray! I felt that this was a real milestone. With the next treatment (the last Taxol treatment), I would be halfway done with my chemo. Time passed slowly as I tried to get through each day. Paul and I stayed active, but we were not busy. We went to MD Anderson often, we saw movies, occasionally we visited with friends, we called friends and family, and I rested a lot. Our life at this time was pretty boring, but that was our life. I wanted very much to get back to living a "normal" life. I wanted to feel good again and to have the energy to do something.

I was physically doing fine. The sores on my head, my arms, and my legs had just about all healed. I still had red spots on my arms and my face, but they were lightening each day. I hoped they would go away soon. My toes were all numb now, and my fingers were all in the process of numbing. I was not as agile on my feet at that time because of my toes, but I walked slowly and tried to be careful. I could still type even though my fingers were numb and that was a good thing. Having fingers that worked meant that I could still write. I had very little hair anywhere on my body. My eyes were now a little less red and sunken.

Fighting fatigue was a constant battle. I spent nearly every evening lying in bed. I purchased (at a garage sale) a bed to put into our living room. Our room looked rather strange with my new small bed, but I felt that the bed was a necessity. We didn't do much entertaining at this time, and I decided style didn't really matter. I had a bed to lie on so that I could watch TV and stay with Paul a little while longer in the evenings. Poor Paul had to do all the physical jobs, and he served as my full-time caregiver. No one ever came to relieve him. I was not good company because I usually did not have the energy to even carry on an enlivened conversation. I just sat and listened. However, I was very lucky. I did not *have* to do anything. Paul kept reminding me that it was all right to not work.

I didn't write much at this time. I did not have the energy to start projects and to finish them. I was not answering e-mails, although I still read and enjoyed them. I remained in physical therapy at MD Anderson and just about had the complete mobility of my arms back. We did leave Houston for two days to drive to Smithville, where we visited with my cousin, Jimmy Neal Stacy and his wife Judy. We enjoyed seeing their home and loved their fresh garden produce. On this trip we also visited with our friends, Cesare and Betty Nadalini. They now live in Tuscany, Italy, in their very own villa. We visited them in their home in Italy in 2002. I worked with Cesare at AT&T and NCR. Betty had ovarian/uterus Cancer in 1994. She had been a help to me during this unplanned journey because she understood what I was going through. She had been a great encouragement to me. We really enjoyed our short visit with these old friends.

Twelfth and Last Taxol Chemo Treatment

On Monday, January 12, 2004, I took my last Taxol chemo treatment. Hooray! Hooray! After this treatment I was fatigued all of the time, except early in the mornings. I wasn't too sick but remained plagued with an aura about me of illness and weakness—I just couldn't really do anything. My toes became even more numb and useless and cold. My fingers also became more numb and asleep—to the point that I cut myself while slicing an onion. I vowed at this point to stop cutting completely until my fingers recovered some. I had this lizardlike condition on both of my hands around my knuckles. My knuckles itched, were red, and felt sore to the touch. They looked like lizard's skin. I finally developed mouth sores. The ulcers that I had with these chemo treatments were a little different from ulcers that I had suffered before Cancer. However despite these new and worsened problems, I felt good that the first regimen of chemo was over.

At this time we were without bicycles so we went out and bought two more bicycles. The apartment complex gave us a storage closet so that we could store our bikes inside this time. Locking them up outside had not been successful in deterring thieves. I hoped that they wouldn't get stolen again. I continued to try to walk and to ride my bike when I could. It was easy to ride the bike or walk trails just across the street from our apartment through Herman Park to MD Anderson.

Even though I had lost quite a bit of weight during these treatments, women on breast Cancer chemo usually gained weight. I had lost down enough that before Christmas, I had bought two pair of size 16 jeans that looked nice on my slimmer figure. I had been a size 18 or a size 20 when I started this battle. I didn't want to gain my weight back. I couldn't figure out how I could gain weight when I felt so bad and was so tired all of the time, but my doctor assured me that I could. So I wanted to exercise as much as I could.

Finding activities that I could do when I was so exhausted took real creativity. I did not enjoy doing my handwork. Before chemo, I was always working on a counted cross-stitch or some handcrafted project. Now my fingers were numb, and my brain didn't have the patience or ability for these handcrafts—I had chemobrain. I did not even like to read very long when I was so fatigued. Reading made me sleepy, and I didn't think that I would be able to sleep all day and then be able to sleep all night also. I wished that I could have been like Rip Van Winkle and just sleep through this entire happening.

The numbness continued to extend further up into my hands and my feet. This is a common side effect of Taxol. At this time, I needed to wear open-toed sandals in order to keep my toes from hurting. I thought that if your toes were numb, you wouldn't be able to feel any pain, but that was not the way that it worked. This kind of numbness actually caused pain. This new pain caused me to be even a little more "out of style" because I now went everywhere in summer sandals even though it was the middle of winter.

The red splotches on my skin began to look a little better. I could not wear eye makeup to cover up my red and sunken eyes because of fears of infection. I had very little hair on my body, but somehow through this entire first ordeal, my eyebrow hairs still stayed firmly attached to their normal place on my face. I had always had dark and rather bushy eyebrows. They weren't so dark now nor were they bushy, but I was thankful for them in a way that I had never been before. They were tough enough to hang on against this powerful Taxol. The one hundred or so hairs that managed to cling to my head looked really funny. I had cut them short to help me in doctoring my head sores, and they were now growing a little longer. I felt lucky to have the stubble. I kept reminding everyone that *"a bad hair day was better than a no-hair day."*

We didn't really do anything to celebrate the end of Taxol. However, we did take a little time off before we started the next chemo regimen, and I received a wonderful gift. I enjoyed a happy, relaxing, laugh-filled weekend and two days away from chemo and from being surrounded by fellow Cancer patients at MD Anderson. I had felt very good during that weekend off—almost normal. Sandra Bradshaw Kurtin, one of my long time friends since early childhood, and her husband, Bill, took us out to spend the weekend in a beach house on the Gulf of Mexico, on Bolivar Peninsula, across from Galveston. We ate gourmet food in seafood restaurants and in Sandra's delicious home cooked meals, we walked on the beach, we talked and laughed, we played adult word games, and we got away from our little apartment in Houston. It was truly a magnificent holiday.

After this last Taxol treatment, I wrote these thoughts in my newsletter:

> My body gets weaker each week from the chemo, but I think that my spirit gets stronger in my battle against Cancer. I continue with my counseling sessions and am deriving more strength through this analysis of my fears, problems, and stresses. Having Cancer causes one to examine life and its meaning, and one is forced to think about life's length or shortness. I had never faced my own mortality before. Because Cancer causes death for so many people, I have faced thoughts about my own death. How would I feel? How would I face the pain? How would my loved ones feel, and how could I help them? What would I leave behind? Would my life have been worthwhile? Will I be strong enough to die with dignity? I had never thought seriously about these questions before. This is truly a time for the evaluation of one's life.

After this enjoyable "gift" weekend, I did not want to go back to MD Anderson that next Wednesday morning of January 21 to begin my next regimen of chemo, but I did.

Chapter 33

Count My Blessings—I'm Alive

I Meet the Red Devil

This new regimen of chemo was very different from the Taxol treatments. I had gone through a "training" session with my doctor the first of January, and I thought that I knew what to expect. I would have to have a blood test that the doctor would review each time before I took the FAC infusion. I was required to see the doctor each time before I actually started the chemo. Each treatment would run on 21 day cycles. We planned to begin my treatments on Wednesday, January 21, 2004, so this would be counted as day one in my 21 day treatment cycle. Each time on day one, I would take a blood test and then go in to see the doctor. If he gave his approval, I would then go to the infusion center and receive the 5 FU drug and the Cytoxan. Then the nurses would start the Adriamycin that must be given continuously over a forty-eight-hour period. They put the Adriamycin in a waist pack pump that I would wear or keep with me for the next forty-eight hours. After getting the waist pack all set up, I would go home and do normal activities with the infusion unit doing its thing from my waist pack. On Friday, after wearing the pump for forty-eight hours, I would come back to the hospital, take off the chemo pump, and receive more infusions of medicines. The actual chemo treatment was over at this time, and I would go home and wait for eighteen more days before beginning the treatment again. I had to go through four of these treatment cycles.

FAC is the chemo that makes you nauseated. To counteract the nausea, the doctors at this time used a drug called Zofran. In 2003, a bottle of thirty of these pills costs $1,280. Fortunately, I had a drug insurance program. My doctor advised me to buy the pills early, and I bought a two-month supply of them in 2003 before my drug program benefits were reduced. My co-pay for each bottle of thirty Zofran pills was $100. I hoped that this supply would last me through my treatments.

The FAC chemo also would hit my white blood cell counts hard so I would have to watch out for infections more carefully than I had done with the Taxol. The doctor planned to monitor my blood counts much more closely than he had done during the Taxol treatments. I understood that I might expect to be sick the first week after the FAC treatment but should to be okay in the second and third weeks.

Hesitation and Fears

I had been given a magnificent respite/holiday from Chemo/Cancer Land. I had spent a delightful weekend with old friends on Galveston Island. My twelfth week of Taxol chemo had gone along uneventfully and had ended on Sunday. I did not go to chemo on Monday. I had a stolen holiday, and it was great. This holiday caused me to wish that I did not have to go to the hospital again. I thought that maybe I did not really have any more Cancer cells in my body. I reasoned in my head that maybe my Cancer had not sent out other Cancer pilgrim cells. Maybe we removed the tumor before it had time to spread. If I were to take the road that I wanted, I would not go back to chemo that Wednesday morning of January 21. I certainly did not want to go, but in reality, I knew that I would pull myself together and walk right back to MD Anderson. Paul insisted that I must do everything possible to reduce the possibility of this Cancer ever reoccurring. He would not let me quit, but it was really, really tempting.

FAC Treatment Number One

Armed with all of this informative information about my new chemo regimen and my expensive antinausea pills, I went to MD Anderson early on the morning of January 21. Blood tests were always performed at eight thirty so that my doctor could get the reports and make his evaluations before my morning appointment. I then went up to see my oncologist, Dr. Brawn. He looked me over and said that everything was okay to start the FAC treatments. I had at this time gained enough weight during the Taxol treatments so that my weight was now the same as it had been before I had my mastectomies. I surely did hate that I had already gained my weight back. In response to my complaints, my wise doctor simply said that a body always seeks "its weight" and that even people who go on a diet and who lose weight usually gain it all back again over time. I didn't like this, but what could I do? I decided that I would just live with my weight gain.

I had developed, of all things, a bladder infection, so Dr. Brawn prescribed amoxicillin for that. With these chemo treatments, I knew that I had to drink lots and lots of water, and I thought that I had. This infection had probably been the cause of the lower-back discomfort that I had felt recently. Dr. Brawn then explained again how I was to take the Zofran, my expensive antinausea pills, and we left the Breast Clinic with another script for medication for my bladder infection and the "hope" that everything coming up would be all right. (Little did I know.)

We then went down to a different transfusion unit—the Bed Transfusion Unit. At this time, there were three separate transfusion units at MD Anderson. As you can probably guess, they administer a lot of chemo. I don't really understand the difference between these areas as they all contain beds. However, this time, I guess that I was under the care of different nurses. I found that mainly Philippine nurses staffed the Bed Transfusion Unit. They had a particular military style about their nursing that I found amusing. They were always in control of the situation. My nurse for that day came in and took me to be weighed. Each time she would send my weight up to the pharmacist who by now had received my chemo orders for the day from my doctor. Using the exact weight that I was on that day, the pharmacist would mix up the bags of medicine that I was to receive and would then send them down to the nurse. Anyway, after my regular weigh in and pressure/temperature check, I got into bed just after noon to begin the second half of my chemotherapy treatments.

The nurse gave me a pill to relax me immediately. I didn't think that I was keyed up, but my blood pressure was 142 when it is normally 110 to 120. The nurse then brought in my IV cocktail packs (bags of medicines). I took a bag of Zofran (the antinausea medicine) first. If a bottle of thirty pills of Zofran costs $1,280, I wondered what a bag of the stuff cost. I would, of course, find out when I got an itemized bill later. Next, I took a bag of 5-Fu and a bag of Cytoxan. I had to eat ice all through the time that I was taking the 5-Fu. It causes sores in your mouth, and the medical people have found that if the patient eats ice during the infusion the occurrence of these mouth sores is reduced. I happily crunched away on my soft ice passing the time. After I had received both the 5-Fu and the Cytoxan, I was done with this first part of my chemo treatment. All of these infusions took about two hours.

The second part of the treatment was to get equipped with the medicine that I would take home with me, the Adriamycin. The nurse brought in a black fanny pack bag and a plastic bag full of red liquid, the Adriamycin. She told me that everyone called this medicine the "Red Devil." She hooked me up to the Adriamycin and let it run for ten minutes to make sure that I suffered no reactions to it. Then she put the red bag of Adriamycin into the fanny pack and taught me how to run the little pump that would control its deliverance. The pump was small like a transistor radio, only thicker. It ran on batteries, was fairly heavy, and was simple to operate. It pumped the Adriamycin into my body very slowly. I took 240 units of this stuff over a forty-eight-hour period. After my "Red Devil" infusion was started and the fanny pack was loaded, I got out of bed, and we left the hospital about 3:00 p.m. This hadn't taken too long, and I felt fine. Maybe my worries were all for naught.

At Home with the Adriamycin Pump

That evening, I had a normal supper and worked some around the house. I wore the pack around my waist and complained that it was really heavy. The night went fine. I took my first Zofran at ten that evening. I had to take them every six to eight hours so I set my alarm and took my second Zofran at 4:00 a.m. I wasn't nauseated, but Paul wanted to make sure that I didn't get that way and insisted that I take my pill on the legal short time allowance. The infusion pack rested on the floor by my bed, with a wire to my body that was long enough to make movement easy while I slept. I had no problems with it, except that I had to remember to pick up the pack when I got up to go to the bathroom during the night. Everything was still fine.

Thursday morning, I got up and ate my normal breakfast of Flax Cereal with a half of banana, sugar, and milk. I worked around the apartment for a few minutes doing morning cleanup chores. However, I quickly decided that I had better go to bed. I took another Zofran at 10:00 a.m. I stayed in bed, dozing in and out of sleep all day, getting sicker as the time passed. Paul had left that morning to go to the apartment office to work doing online trading just before I had started to feel sick. Pyewacken (a new cat in our family, whose story will be written later) and I lay on the bed all day. I didn't eat or drink anything because I was becoming more nauseated each hour.

About 2:00 p.m., my cycle of continual vomiting began. My stomach had always been the "weak" part of my body. I had always been susceptible to throwing up. Earlier in my life I had thrown up in cars, planes, and boats. I threw up and gagged when anyone else threw up—even my own children. I threw up when I got an acid stomach. It wasn't difficult for me to throw up. However, usually immediately after I threw up, the feeling of nausea went away, and I felt better. But with this chemo nausea, a vomiting spell did not give me that same feeling of relief. After each of these spells, I went back to bed and felt just as nauseated and miserable as I had before I vomited. There was *no* relief from it. When I had suffered from motion sickness, the feeling of nausea was similar, but I knew that the second I stepped onto land off a boat, the feeling of sickness would leave instantly. I didn't know where the "land" was in this sickness, and I had no way of knowing how to find it and to make the nausea go away.

Paul came home from his financial work to find me still vomiting even though I ate or drank nothing. The Zofran pills would calm my stomach for about two and a half hours, and then the nausea would rage again. I would throw up even though I had nothing but stomach bile to retch. I thought that my toes were going to curl up and come out of my mouth. I would get hot, vomit, and become completely wet all over with sweat. After I could stop retching, I was, of course, freezing and shaking from the cooling sweat that was all over my body. At about 10:00 p.m., after I had thrown up one of those forty-three-dollar pills, we decided to call the Triage Nursing Center at MD Anderson. (I couldn't even keep the antinausea medicine in my stomach.) Triage advised me to let the Zofran melt in my mouth and not to take *any* water. So I did. I went on my *no nothing* by mouth regimen. I took my Zofran every six hours as it was prescribed. I would vomit regularly, but I did manage to sleep in between the spells. Thank God for these small blessings of rest.

The next morning, the vomiting continued. The Jell-O that I had wanted the evening before had jelled overnight, and I ate two tablespoons of it for breakfast. I ate two ice cubes. Nothing stayed down. I retched and vomited and retched again. All of this time, I felt like dying would be a blessing and a relief. There didn't seem to be anything that would help my immediate sufferings here on earth. The pump continued to deliver the "Red Devil" into my body. I wished that I could rip that pump off and run far, far away, never to do this awful thing to my body again, but I didn't.

About 11:00 a.m., Paul could stand no more of my distress and called my doctor. My doctor prescribed another medication, ABH. When asked whether I wanted this in pill form or in suppository form, I chose the suppository because I didn't think that I could keep down a pill. I managed to get a bath before we had to go back to MD Anderson for the next part of my treatment. It was nearing the time that the Adriamycin would be all finished. I was *so* very sick. I had not eaten or drunk anything that stayed on my stomach for more than a few minutes in the past thirty-six hours.

Back to the Hospital for the Final Infusions

I managed to walk into the hospital with my trash-can vomit receptacle while tears were just a breath way. Crying at this stage was the normal status for me. I went into the public at the hospital and hated to have everyone seeing me crying. But fortunately, the public at MD Anderson was full of Cancer patients, Cancer patient nurses, receptionists, or other people very involved with Cancer on a daily basis. Thank goodness. Everyone was very understanding and kind. I found my way to the Infusion Bed Unit and signed in while Paul parked our car. We normally parked the car in the garage and walked into the hospital together, but today, I did not have the strength to walk that far.

We were about twenty minutes early, and the waiting room was full. There is always at least one couch in each waiting area, and two ladies seeing my state of sickness graciously got up and gave me a couch so that I could lie down. The receptionist brought me out a pillow. I waited lying down with my vomit trash can nearby. About 2:20 p.m., I went back into the infusion unit. I went through the usual weigh-in on the same scale that I had weighed on exactly forty-eight hours earlier. In this forty-eight-hour period of chemo, I had lost nine pounds; The "Red Devil" poison had done "a deed" on me. My blood pressure was 156 over 88, which is *very* high for me, and my temperature was 99.4, which is over two degrees higher than my normal temperature of 97. I no sooner got into my bed than I proceeded to vomit again—nothing but stomach bile.

The Philippine nurse came in, saw me, and started to fuss. She said, "Why didn't you come into the emergency room? You could have become dehydrated? You have made yourself sore and weak. Why did you do this?" I told her that I didn't think that vomiting was a condition that warranted ER treatment. She told me that I was wrong. Anyway, she set up my medicines, and just on time, my pump signaled that my Adriamycin infusion was complete.

At about that time, another nurse came in and exclaimed, "What is wrong with your face? What has been happening to you?" Now you must remember this group of nurses is a corps of Philippine nurses complete with accents, strict discipline, and commanding methods. I looked up at her and thought maybe I had all of a sudden grown two noses. I really hadn't looked at myself in the mirror during this vomiting episode so I didn't really know what was wrong with my face. I asked Paul, and he told me that my face was very flushed. After a little more ranting, the second nurse left the room, and I vowed as soon as I got to a mirror that I would "check out" my face one more time.

But now the Adriamycin infusion was complete. I was really glad of that! The nurse took off the "Red Devil" pack. She flushed my line and gave me another bag of Zofran. To complete this treatment, I received another bag of 5-Fu, although this time, I didn't eat ice through the infusion. I was too nauseated. I completed the treatment by taking the whole bag of saline because I felt that I needed the fluid. We finished at the hospital about 4:00 p.m. and went home. I was still sick and nauseated, but I was relieved to be done with this first FAC treatment. I think that the "Red Devil" had won this round, and I was completely defeated. What was I going to do? How would I ever be able to stand three more of these "treatments" that were a living Hell on earth?

At home, I took the ATH (my new antinausea medicine, which I had chosen to get in pill form) and tried to settle down. I was still taking the Zofran every six hours. My infusion nurse had advised me to eat even though I was nauseated. About 6:00 p.m., even though I had taken the extra medicine, I vomited again. After this episode, however, I decided to eat a poached egg and a piece of dry toast. The first food that had passed my lips in three days tasted good. My infusion nurse had told me that it was better to have something in my stomach to throw up than it was to keep throwing up just stomach bile. However, after this small meal, I got nauseated again. I lay in bed with cold rags on my face and neck, trying to keep something down. I took another ATH at 10:00 p.m. and waited for the medicine to calm my raging stomach. With much careful work, I managed to keep this egg down and went to sleep for a good night's rest.

Paul woke me up at 2:00 a.m. to take another Zofran. I went back to sleep and woke up again at 7:30 a.m. The nightmare seemed to be over. My extreme and continuous nausea was gone. It was pouring down rain outside, but the sun was shining on my spirit. I got up and ate my Flax Cereal breakfast and rested. I continued take the Zofran for twenty-four hours more, interspersed with the new antinausea medicine ATH, but hopefully, the really bad part of this chemo treatment was over. I wondered what chemo treatments were like before they had the super antinausea medicines. I shuddered to think of it.

Thoughts about Cancer

Cancer is a powerful and dreadful disease that affects everyone around it in an unforgettable way. I didn't at the time really understand how it had affected me, but I did know that I would be changed forever when I got through this unplanned journey. Many, many people fight this Cancer battle over and over again. I hadn't begun to pray that I did not have to fight this battle again, but I would begin to pray that prayer soon. I was continually amazed at the courage that people have when three, six, or even ten years later, they find another Cancer in their bodies. I ran into these people every day at MD Anderson. They were usually happy and calm and optimistic. They somehow managed to take on each battle against this disease thinking that the outcome would be a good one. They demonstrated a courage that I had never seen up close before.

When I realized that I was becoming a part of this population of Cancer-fighting people, I was forced to be strong and courageous also—sometimes when I certainly didn't really feel that way.

Alive to Go On

In the meantime, the worst of my first FAC chemo treatments was over. I thanked God! Next time, I would be more knowledgeable about what to do and what not to do. I would be armed with a second antinausea drug. I certainly did not like taking all of this medicine but I now felt that I really needed all of it. If there was any way that I could stop these treatments, I would. I hadn't talked to Mary Joy about stopping, but Paul would not hear of me quitting. He didn't want me to have Cancer again and felt that the best way for me to ensure not having Cancer again was to take the recommended preventative measures—one of the biggest of these was chemotherapy. I did decide that chemotherapy drugs were probably what Satan used to attack poor old Job's body back in the Old Testament. The description of what plagues Satan sent on Job sounded a lot like the symptoms of my chemo drugs.

How the mind does play with images when it has lots of time! I was passing time just waiting for the chemo treatments to be over. I still had very numb fingers and toes. I had one sore (ulcer) in my mouth that just wouldn't heal. I still had red spots all over my arms and a remaining few on my legs. However, they seemed to be improving. I thought that since I was now off of the Taxol, the strange-looking sores that had been on my legs since the beginning of Taxol would finally heal. My lizard hands were peeling and seemed to be getting a little better. I was afraid that I might lose even more of the few hairs that I had with this FAC. No one would predict how each chemo would affect each patient. My fatigue level seemed to be better. I was regularly riding my bike back and forth to MD Anderson.

I talked to my "support team" through my regular and long newsletters. This is what I wrote after my first FAC treatment:

> Time goes slowly, but it does pass. Before I know it, I hope, it will be spring again. I only have three more treatments of FAC to take, and I have the free time of two weeks before I have to take the second dose. I take the next treatment on February 11. The doctor will not schedule any more than the next one of these treatments because he will have to watch my bloodwork to keep me from getting too "down." Continue, please, to pray and hope that these Cancer drugs that are in my body will kill any

and all Cancer cells there and, at the same time, will not hurt any of the organs or good parts of my body. God has kept his hand on me throughout this battle, and I am sure that he will continue to do so. After all, I have the best "support" group that any person could have. I am lucky and blessed.

I must never forget to *always "count my blessings."* The first of my four FAC treatments was over, and I was alive.

Chapter 34

KEEPING ON KEEPING ON

A Time between Treatments

The first treatment of my new chemo regimen was over, and things started getting better each day. My tastes began to come back. I was only nauseated occasionally. I ate nothing but homemade chicken noodle soup for two days after the horrible forty-eight-hour nausea experience that I had. A good friend of mine, (the mother of number one son's wife, Liz), brought over a frozen batch of her homemade chicken noodle soup. It saved my life. It was very rich and thick and tasty. I lived off of this gourmet delight while my taste and smell were messed up with chemo. It was the only food that I found tolerable.

However, five days into this first chemo cycle, I could actually eat a nearly normal meal. I had about three bites of meat and lots of fresh vegetables. They were my own special kind of vegetables—turnip greens, stewed okra, cucumbers in rice vinegar, and fresh tomato slices, but they were at least more than chicken noodle soup. I experienced a little nausea now and then, but I had not actually vomited since I had taken the "red devil" 48-hour chemo treatment. I was recovering from the first FAC treatment. I had only three more treatments to go. Thank God!

My time "resting" after the first FAC treatment was a good time. My energy level began to increase. My body was enjoying the "rest" time. My skin was finally really getting better. My eyes were not so horribly red and sunken. My skin was healing and began to look nearly normal. I still had purple "scars" from each of the Taxol sores, but hopefully they would disappear in time. I still had a few red splotches on my arms, but they were also getting better.

I now had *no* hair anywhere. My eyebrows, which had managed to hang on all through Taxol, had finally given up the ghost and were nearly all gone. I didn't have any eyelashes at this time either. In fact, I don't think that I had a single hair left on my body. I worked hard expanding my hat and colored headband wardrobe. I wore my favorite Cancer hat (a cream-colored straw) with a colored hatband that I changed with each outfit. I actually received compliments on this hat even though I knew that hats weren't really in style. I liked wearing my Cancer hat, and it seemed to look good on my bald head with some type of knit cap underneath covering my baldness.

I did have a reoccurrence of a bladder infection and increased neuropathy, but my physical condition was good. And for just having compleated a chemo treatment, I was feeling *very* well.

FAC Treatment a Second Time

I managed to get through the second chemo FAC treatment easier. This time, my doctor doubled the amount of Zofran (the really expensive antinausea drug), which he gave me in the IV. He also added Zofran in the backpack of Adriamycin that I took for forty-eight hours. In addition I took an antinausea pill every four hours (one time, I would take Zofran, and the next time, I would take ABH), and of course, I got another dose of Zofran when I went in to take my final portion of this treatment. This time, I was not so nauseated. I threw up only twice during this round of chemo. However, I still lost five pounds in forty-eight hours. I can't really figure out how I lost this much weight because I didn't vomit nor did I have diarrhea. I didn't exercise either—I didn't feel good and just lay around in bed.

In my newsletter that I wrote at this time, I expressed feelings of discouragement even as I laughed at my condition:

> This Cancer is just *not* a winning battle anyway that you go. I thought that while I was way off by myself (away from all my old friends), I would perform an "extreme makeover." You know, lose weight, grow curly luxurious hair, etc. However, it looks like I am not going to lose weight, and I have no hair so I guess I should just give up on the "extreme makeover." I have decided to just *get through this time.* I will lose weight later, and hopefully I will grow some kind of hair again. After having had no hair, I will be happy with whatever color or kind of hair that grows in. Anyway, I now only have two more chemo treatments to go. Hooray! Hooray!

> While I go down this Cancer road, I am getting another lesson in understanding and tolerance. This time it is *don't criticize anyone else for doing something that seems to be stupid. You don't know how they feel unless you have walked in their shoes.* I should have learned this somewhere before, but I think that I must have forgotten it. I will remember this important lesson now the rest of my life. I could never understand why patients who were critically ill could ever stop taking their medicines. Well, now I think I have some idea about why they do this. I have become a pill junky. During my last chemo treatment, I was taking seven different

types of pills. I was taking two antinausea pills—alternating one every four hours. I was taking Cipro, an antibiotic that I was taking for my persistent bladder infection. This medicine had to be taken twice a day on an empty stomach, which meant I had to take it two hours after eating and two hours before I ate again. I had to be sure to drink a big glass of water with this pill. I was taking another bladder pill that turns my urine bright orange. (At this time I surely had the gaudiest pee in the neighborhood.) This pill had to be taken three times a day, which means in eight-hour intervals, with food. I am taking Neurontin to help the neuropathy (numbness in my fingers, toes, and feet). I am now taking three of these 100 mg pills in a dose. Each dose should be taken three times a day. I am taking Lexapro for depression. I take it one time a day, just before I go to bed. (It is a simple pill.) And finally, I take Prilosec for my reflux. It must be taken in the morning, thirty minutes before I eat anything. What a regimen it is to keep all of these pills straight!

I think that one must be a genius in order to take all of these pills correctly all of the time. Paul joined in to help me run this, scheduling my pill-taking project. I first made a daily chart with the times written down as to when I was going to take each pill in a time-sequenced order. We made a check notation when I had taken each pill and corrected the time if we were late or early in taking it. What a pain! I can now swallow four pills in one big gulp. It always amazed me that my mother could swallow a handful of pills in one swallow. I thought that I could never do this, but I can. It is amazing what one learns when one suddenly finds himself in different situations. Anyway, through all of this, I have gained an understanding as to why some chronic patients with diseases like bipolar disorders can stop taking their pills. If I forget or get lazy and do not eat something with the pill that requires food, I get sick and vomit. I then have the dilemma of trying to decide whether to take the medicines again or whether I should just wait until they are due again. How can I know if I vomit one and one-half hours after taking a pill, whether I have gotten the medicine absorbed into my body or not? I don't know, and I feel awful for several hours from the vomiting spell. I am sure that the chemo that I am taking, Adriamycin (the "Red Devil"), accentuates the nausea. I feel that I am much more vulnerable to this condition right now than when I am in a normal body state. Anyway, I now hate to take pills and would throw them all out the window, except that I know that I can't. However, I always try to remember that *this (chemo time) shall pass!* Dear God, I think that I have *really* learned this lesson. I will be understanding of others now even when what they do seems crazy to me. I promise that I will never again get upset when someone else stops taking his or her pills.

Food and FAC

After this second treatment, I still very much depended on the homemade chicken noodle soup as my main food for several days after the chemo treatment was finished. I had eaten all of the batch that was given to me after the first treatment. However, Liz Dittmer, number one son's wife, got the recipe from her mother and made another recipe of the soup for me. It seemed to help settle my nausea and satisfied my hunger when nothing else smelled or sounded good. I enjoyed Liz's soup this time and was able to freeze most of it so that I could continue to eat it throughout these treatments. Liz had given me the recipe. It was the best soup for an upset stomach that I have ever found, and it was delicious.

When I walked by the MD Anderson Cafeteria the smells wafting out of the prepared foods was always delicious and inviting. It was a very good cafeteria. However, after this second FAC treatment, the smell in the hallway nearly made me throw up. *Chemo does strange things to your sense of smell and taste.*

Holiday Celebrations

It was strange, but Paul and I did not really celebrate holidays during this year of Cancer. It was not anything that we ever talked about. We had gone through the Fourth of July, Halloween, Thanksgiving, my birthday, Christmas, Paul's birthday, and now Valentine's Day. Neither of us had really celebrated any of these holidays. We went through the motions. I bought Paul an electric razor for Christmas. I baked him a birthday cake. I gave Christmas presents to the family and to our friends. However, Paul and I have not exchanged a card or held a single celebration ourselves for any of these holidays. We didn't even exchange Valentine's card. I received several beautiful Valentine cards from friends and supporters, and I thoroughly enjoyed them. We ate Thanksgiving dinner with our son Peter and his family. We went to the family Christmas party. Holidays just didn't seem to be that important compared to the battle that we were fighting against Cancer. I wouldn't have noticed this oddity with a single holiday, but as the holidays came and went, a definite pattern was clear. Easter was coming in a couple of weeks after I took my last chemo treatment. I hoped that by then, maybe we would feel like celebrating again. Maybe we would begin to celebrate holidays again with the celebration of Easter, 2004, which I hoped would represent the end of my year of Cancer.

Paul and I grew very close through this experience. He didn't really feel the suffering that I had to endure, but he nearly felt it. I know now that when I cried telling someone about my difficulties, he cried too. Men do not cry easily, but he was so close to me that he sympathetically felt my pain and cried a few tears when he saw me cry. I knew that he would change things for me if he could, but he couldn't. He continued to care for me diligently each day. I wrote my thanks again and again for the continued prayers and support of my "support team." This year of

Cancer had been an earth-shattering experience in our lives. It had affected my whole family and even my friends. I hoped that it had affected everyone in a positive way. I was at this time still too close to the experience to judge, but now I feel that my Cancer affected people in a good way. If this book is successful, it will open doors for me to tell my story and to make women aware that they must religiously do a monthly self-breast exam. I think that the things I learned in my unplanned journey will help other Cancer patients. I started to end all of my newsletters in a new way. Read what I wrote in the following newsletter closing to my friends and supporters:

> Take care of yourself and your loved ones. Do your monthly self-breast exam and be diligent about finding Cancer. Remember, *Cancer is curable if it is found early.* They do miracles here a MD Anderson, but people also die here. Cancer is real and *very* dangerous.

Fingernail and Toenail Infections

One day, I noticed that my fingernails and toenails were dark purple and dead yellow. My nails had pulled away from the nail bed. I wondered if they would fall off. I had to be very careful and to not hit or to pull on these nails. The ends of my fingers hurt if they hit anything. My big toenails oozed and looked like they were dead things that were rotting. When I showed my nail condition to my doctor, he told me to go home and to cut the nails off as short as I could. He gave me another antibiotic to take for this new infection. The infection seemed to get better, but my thumbnail was still running stinky gunk. I had to soak it in vinegar and water in order to control the smell.

My right toenail loosened nearly all the way to the back of the nail. Before I could cut my toenails completely off, Paul while asleep in our bed accidentally kicked my right big toe and knocked the nail off. It surely did hurt, but now I didn't have to try to cut it. I tried to think that things could be worse, although sometimes I wondered just how. I really looked strange now without fingernails or toenails, and I was further handicapped. I hadn't realized how often you use your fingernails to do so many daily tasks. But eventually, my nails grew back. My fingernails grew back very quickly as soon as I finished the FAC. However, after five years, my two big toenails are just about to be normal again. Apparently, toenails grow back very slowly.

Neuropathy

My neuropathy remained a real problem. It had gotten worse not better, even though it had now been four weeks since I had received Taxol. My nurse indicated that the other chemo drugs supported the atrophy that first caused the numbness and that probably, the numbness in my fingers and in my feet would not go away until after all the chemo was over. I did get a medicine that helped the neuropathy (Neurontin). It dialed the numbness in my hands back enough that I could make a fist and type. The numbness in my feet had gone back to the ball of my foot so that half of my foot was without feeling. Balancing became difficult, and I was no longer sure-footed. I had to be careful not to fall. It felt like my toes had a rolled-up piece of material under each one. They felt like they were swollen, even though they were not. It was hard to move them. They felt like they were cold all of the time. I had to wear shoes that had ample toe room. If I stood up on the balls of my feet, I was in real danger of falling down because the balls of my feet had no feeling in them. I had trouble using the pedal on the piano, the pedal on my sewing machine, and the gas pedal on the car. But even with the medicine, the neuropathy in my hands remained a big problem. I could not open pop-top cans. I could not button and unbutton small buttons. If anything hard hit the ends of my fingers, they hurt. I was not sure in cutting things with a knife and had to be very careful that I did not cut my hands. I couldn't push anything in that was hard to push.

I refused to lose my ability to type (write). Typing felt funny right at that time, and I often got off onto the wrong keys, but I continued to write. My typing was terrible. However, I was patient even though I had to go back and do a lot of correcting. Paul always checked my writing also, so hopefully I didn't send out too many mistakes. However, even if it was more difficult, my writing was an outlet for me that I used to help me keep my sanity. I promised my readers that I would continue to send my newsletters throughout this disease even if I had to dictate them, and have Paul type them. However, I was always able to type and kept doing my writing.

Finding handwork that I could do was really hard. I tried putting together puzzles to fill the time in the evenings when we sat and watched TV. I was never a good sitter. I had to be doing something with my hands in order to keep my mind satisfied. Watching TV by itself was not enough. I couldn't do my counted cross-stitch. It was much too difficult for my mind and my numb fingers. I couldn't embroider because it was hard to hold a tiny needle with my numb fingers. I was lost for a while, searching for something that I could do. Then one morning, while watching the *Martha Stewart* show, I got an idea. She suggested a good use for the beautiful wool men's suits that men no longer wear. She suggested that we make quilted wraps from these lovely materials. I didn't want to make wraps, but I did think that I could make a beautiful quilt from these no longer needed or old and worn items of clothing.

So I began collecting (buying cheaply) at garage sales and thrift stores suits, jackets, even a skirt or two made of beautiful wool fabrics. I brought these "out of fashion" items of clothing home and ripped them apart. I could sit at the TV and break the article down to its pieces. I then pressed these pieces with a steam iron and rolled them into bundles that I would later cut into squares to sew together into a quilt when my neuropathy got better. I had finally found an activity that I could do to keep me busy and happy during this last part of chemo. I was planning to make my Cancer Quilt. I was sure that it would be very warm and interesting. It would always remind me of the time when my hands didn't work well.

My counselor pointed out that this quilt-making activity ran parallel to what was happening in my life. She pointed out that with the effects of the Cancer and my works in sorting out my inner thoughts, fears, and feelings, I was tearing my life all apart, evaluating each section, and that I would eventually sew it all back together again. I was looking at all the basic parts of my life, all the things that I had accepted as "truth" without even thinking of it before, and now I was examining and ripping each "truth" apart and rearranging things, discarding the "disguised untruths" and coming up with a totally new set of values and realities—a new life standard that would be symbolized by my wool quilt. She said that this activity was a real symbol of my unplanned journey.

I don't know that I totally believed all of the symbolisms that she drew from my quilt. However, the quilt-making activities were very helpful to me. I have not yet finished the quilt. I have all of these nice four-inch-square blocks of different wool materials sorted, organized, bagged, and stored in the top of my closet. I hope that I have rearranged the "truths" in my life and have gone on. Maybe the writing of this book is the symbolic "putting together" of my life's values. Someday I will slow down long enough to concentrate on sewing these pieces into my quilt. Right now, this book is the putting together of my new life standards from having experienced this unplanned journey (my Cancer fight).

All of these new handicaps really made me glad that Paul was with me all of the time. I didn't do a lot of my tasks in my normal fashion anymore, but I tried very hard to still do as much as I could. I never mentioned the accelerator pedal problem to Paul or to my doctors. I surely didn't want to lose my driving privileges even though some of the medicines that I took did preclude my driving. Paul drove me nearly everywhere that I went, but I didn't want to ever become completely dependent on someone else. I didn't ever want to lose my "freedom."

Thoughts on Taking the Next Treatment

I had my third FAC treatment scheduled for March 8, 9, and 10. I hated the thought of taking the chemo. I now knew that it was tough taking the chemicals for three days, but when it was finished, so far I had recovered quickly. I thought that the extreme nausea was now under control also. And I remembered that the good thing was that after this treatment, I only had to take one more. Hooray! Hooray! I was nearly finished!

During this time, I had fears of taking the next round of chemo. The following is an excerpt from one of my letters at the time:

I would like to run away and *not* take the next chemo, but I will not do that. I will finish the job that I started, but I wish that I could run away and wouldn't have to think about Cancer ever again. Maybe this time I can get control of the nausea so that my experience isn't so bad. I do think that I will go to the ER this time if the vomiting is like it was with the first treatment.

Trip Back to Grapevine

I would like to tell you this story in my own words as I wrote them at the time so I will again quote from my newsletter:

We went to church at our home church, Living Word Lutheran Church, in Grapevine. We have been going to this church for eighteen years and have been very active. I walked in and passed friends of mine in the Bell Choir (that I had played with for years), and these friends looked at me and didn't recognize me. I had to tell them to stop and to look at me again. Then they recognized me and were glad to see me. We enjoyed seeing our old friends. I wore my dark wig that day, and everyone told me that I looked great. Of course, I always felt like they were just being kind. The fact that they didn't recognize me told me volumes about the way that I looked!

When I look into the mirror right now, I don't recognize myself. I don't feel on the inside like I look on the outside. I never knew before what my head was shaped like. It was always covered with hair. I had really never thought about how I would look without hair. I believe that my face must be swollen a little from the steroids that I have been taking with the chemo. That may be the reason that my eyes look so sunken. I continue to be ugly, ugly, ugly. I hope that this is a temporary condition. I hope that I will be well and strong and vibrant again soon.

I must add that Paul does not think that I am ugly. He is adamant about this. He always reads and proofs my writings and sometimes has his own comments. He insisted that I tell you that he does not feel like I do. He thinks that I look different during Cancer, but to him, I am not ugly. That is true love, don't you think?

One of my old friends from our Grapevine church had had breast Cancer in the early 1990s. She had told me about her Cancer experience and about how bad her chemo had been, but she had assured me that I could do it. She hadn't, however, told me that she had quit her chemo before her regimen had ended. Her husband related this story to Paul privately that Sunday when we were visiting. What a surprise! She had not indicated to me in any way that she hadn't finished her chemo. Apparently, she was all right now since it had been many years since she had had Cancer. But I guess there really are people who quit this awful stuff. I thought long and hard about this story and wished that I could quit. *Chemo has to be the worst "good" thing that you can do to your body.*

MD Anderson Thoughts

Facing my own death was something that I couldn't help but think about at this time. I expressed some of these thoughts in my letters as follows:

When one walks around MD Anderson all of the time, you can't help but think and ask the question, "When is the time to die?" I see old people there who are so sick and weak. I don't know that I would have the strength to fight Cancer in their condition. I think that I might be tempted to say, "I've had a good life. Maybe it is time for me just to quit and to die." I wonder if I would have the courage and the wisdom to make that decision. Would I hurt or help my children if I made that decision? I definitely do not want to die from Cancer. I now look on dying differently than I did before. My father died of a stroke one day when he was 64. My brother was killed instantly in a car wreck when he was 65. (He had just retired from his high school counseling job.) Both of these deaths were a great shock to the family and me. However, now I think that my father and my brother were lucky. They both died quickly and "easily" while they were strong and still working. These were good ways to die. I hope that I can die in a similar manner. I do not want to be sick and to be an invalid for a long period of time. How sad are some of these people who are patients at MD Anderson! It takes a strong person to be at MD Anderson.

I often wanted to run away somewhere and to just forget all about Cancer. But I didn't. *I held fast to the fact that each day, near my apartment, the bayou kept running to the sea and the sun kept rising and setting, and I knew that I too would continue on this road that I had started (chemo), although it certainly was something that I really did not want to do.*

Valentine Wishes for My Family and Friends

Paul and I weren't really celebrating the holidays, but I knew that everyone else was, and I wrote a Valentine's wish for my team of supporters. It is quoted from my letter dated February 10, 2004, as follows:

BREAST CANCER: THE UNPLANNED JOURNEY - LESSONS LEARNED

I wish each of you a happy Valentine's Day. Enjoy your loves whether they are old or young. *Love is the grease that keeps the life machine going.* If it weren't for our loving, we wouldn't have a reason to get up each morning and to do our work. Our loved ones make life worth living. How could we get along without them? I certainly couldn't get along without the tons of love and support that I have received during this unplanned journey. And of course, I couldn't do it without the love and support of my love, Paul. May your lives be filled abundantly with love.

Chapter 35

THE END OF THE JOURNEY

The Third Treatment

I got through the third FAC chemo treatment on March 8 without incident. The treatments were never fun, but I now knew that I could do them. This treatment made me feel sick, but I didn't ever throw up. Thoughts of certain things and smells could make me instantly nauseous. I felt sure that the threatening spells of nausea would go away as I got further out in time from the treatment. I only lost two pounds this time during the chemo treatment.

My skin started to show real improvement. I still had a few scars and blotches, but they were steadily getting lighter. My skin was softening and getting closer to normal also. My eyes were no longer red and sunken. My toes were still plagued with numbness. I needed to be walking a lot, and it just wasn't fun to walk with my toes flapping on the end of my feet. However, overall, I was doing very well. My energy level was good, and after the first week after the treatment, I wasn't sick.

Finally, New Hair

Eight days after this third treatment, I noticed that the top of my head felt funny. Somehow, it just didn't feel the same as it had felt. I rubbed it and rubbed it all day long, thinking to myself, "What in the world is wrong with my head?" It no longer felt smooth. By evening, I took the time to go into the bathroom and took a good look in the mirror. I was very surprised to see that I was growing fuzz on my head. I was exhilarated! This was a sure sign that the end was near and that I really was going to return to "normal" again someday. Hallelujah! The flowers were blooming everywhere outside, and my hair decided to sprout also! I ran in to have Paul feel my new fuzz. He simply said, "Don't get too excited yet. You can hardly even see the fuzz." I was excited anyway. I didn't have enough hair to blow in the wind, but I did have some fuzz to flutter in a breeze. I was very happy!

Fourth FAC Treatment

Blood Count Too Low

I went to the hospital on schedule on Wednesday, March 29, to get my last chemo treatment. I had gone the night before to have my blood tested. Just as I had done for the prior six months, I went in to see the doctor to have a short checkup visit. To my complete surprise, he told me that I could not take chemo that day. My blood counts were too low. I felt fine and I had trouble understanding why my blood counts were so low. He scheduled my treatment for the next week and told me to go home and rest. That was good in that now I didn't have to take the treatment, but it was bad because I had to wait a week in order to finish. This had thrown my carefully drawn X-off chart off. Now I had to figure out how to wait. I had never been very good at just waiting.

Friends Come to Help Pass the Weekend

However, two of my very best girlfriends, Sharon Reynolds Kimbrell and Barrilyn Gorman Roberts, came to visit that weekend. What a wonderful time we had! Two of my other special classmates from McCamey High School came on Saturday afternoon to join us, Miles and Linda Lou McDonald. Poor Paul was overwhelmed, I think. But we all just talked and talked and laughed and laughed. It was amazing that such old friends could be such good friends even after fifty years. *Friends are one of the sweetest things in life.*

That evening at dinner, we toasted to the fact that you didn't get the chance to choose your family, but you did get to choose your friends. We chose each other and are very happy for it. I wore myself to a frazzle that weekend, but I really did have a super good time. It helped me pass the time before my final chemo treatment. Paul and I took Barri and Sharon to the airport on Sunday morning, came home, and then went to church. After church, I went to bed and slept the rest of the day. Before I had time to get worried about the fourth treatment, it was Monday morning and time to go to the hospital. I was so grateful to my friends for giving me such a fun filled, busy weekend.

Finally I Get the Last FAC Treatment

I was finally able to take my final FAC treatment on Monday, April 5. The infusion was uneventful, except that I ran a fever that Sunday, Monday, and Tuesday. I think that the weekend with my friends tired me more than I realized. However, I took the IV drugs. I took the antinausea pills. I felt bad. I rested and then on Wednesday, April 7, I went back to the hospital to take off the infusion backpack and to take my final IV chemo. They took out my central line port from my chest after I had completed this treatment. I was done! Life could begin again!

The Natural High (written 4:10 a.m. early Thursday)

The best way to tell you how I felt after the last chemo infusion was completed is to quote directly from my writing at the time. A long excerpt from one of my letters written at this time follows:

> How does one explain what it feels like to be done with the treatment of Cancer? You know what the lead shield bib feels like that you put on in the dentist's chair before you have x-rays taken of your mouth? You know the time that the technician sets the machine to go off and runs out of the room, leaving you all weighted down in the chair? I feel like a coat made out of that lead that weighs nearly a ton has been lifted from my body. I feel the beginnings of freedom. I know that I still have to survive this last treatment and to absorb all of the side effects that it may have on my body, but I know now that when I begin to get well from this treatment, I will no longer have to go back to MD Anderson and take another round of that devastating medicine. Hurray! Hurray! Hurray! I can hardly believe that the Cancer and the treatment for it are finally over. When I found out that I had Cancer, I didn't know whether I could really pick my body up and "do" this disease from beginning to end. I didn't know whether I had the strength to endure the "cure." As I got into the treatments, and they became a fact of life, I still didn't know whether I could tolerate all of them. But somehow, with all of your continuous encouragements; the wonderful, loving support of my caregiver, Paul; and God's strength and care; I did it. I completed the unplanned journey! I fought the faithful fight. I endured gracefully. And now it is all over.
>
> Life can begin again. *And oh, how sweet life is!* Cancer has taught me a limited amount of patience. I don't mind waiting in lines or for appointments as I did before. I no longer get irritated if Paul makes a wrong turn when I just told him the right way to go. I no longer find myself getting angry about being caught in traffic or by getting cut off by and aggressive driver. *The effects of my Cancer have changed me . . .*
>
> I am facing a new life (or the reopening of my old life), with only about a fourth inch of fuzz on my head. My fingernails are cut back to within three-eighths of an inch from the place that they start to grow out of my fingers. My toes are numb. The tips of my fingers are numb and sensitive since I don't have much fingernail to protect them. My skin is actually clearing up and looking much better now. I have no breasts.

I am weak and out of shape. I am awkward and in no way the sure-footed athlete that I was when I started this ordeal last July. I am the same weight that I started this whole Cancer thing at. I know that I must look ugly, but I really don't care. *I am very happy to be alive and to not have Cancer in my body. Hallelujah!*

I felt a *big* natural high, a sense of accomplishment having completed the most difficult task that I had attempted ever before in my life. I felt an optimism that would carry me through several years of daily stresses. This long and difficult unplanned journey was finally over! My life could now go on normally.

Let me tell you about the events of my life then and the marvelous world that I found myself in immediately after chemo. Of course, it was spring both in Houston and in Grapevine. The geraniums that we had carefully saved over the winter that we hauled to Houston last October from Grapevine burst from their winter dormancy with about a half dozen beautiful red flower blooms, with more coming each day. These red splendents brightened our little back porch with their gorgeous flaming blossoms that didn't wilt or die for weeks.

The blooms of the azaleas in Houston were tired now and were on their last legs, but the bougainvilleas were blooming along with the redbuds, the fruitless peach trees, the hibiscus, and many other summer flowers. The roadsides along Interstate I-45 were delightful on our drive back to Grapevine. The bluebonnets south of Corsicana were in full bloom and, since we had had a wet winter, were quite lush. The roadways were abounding with Indian paintbrush, pink buttercups, a tall light blue lacy flower, a ten-inch-high yellow-looking daisy with flowers that are about two inches in width, and lots of other small wild flowers. The grasses were full and dark green. This was a bountiful spring that promised to open the door for a bountiful summer in the South just as the end of chemo promised to open the door to a new, bright, full, and rich life for me. I would fly again!

Beginning Life Again

I endured the same usual symptoms immediately after this last infusion—nausea from smells, aching joints, and a little diarrhea. The worst side effect was that the fuzz on the top of my head all fell out. I was bald again.

We left Houston for a visit back to Grapevine on Friday, April 9. I wanted to spend Easter with our family. We had a family lunch in Granbury at Paul Damian's house (number six son), with eight of our grandchildren present. We had a traditional Easter egg hunt (inside) because it was cold and raining outside. The bad weather could not dampen my spirits. I read the grandkids the final edition of *Flat Stanley's Adventures with Grandmother B, Part 2*. This is the second of the children's books that I had written during this unplanned journey.

That evening, I attended a three-hour Catholic baptism and confirmation service for my son, John (number five son). John joined his wife and family by uniting with them at church.

It was a moving ceremony. I held up physically through the long service and the celebration afterward. My knee nearly got me down as the evening progressed, but I trudged on limping around slowly on John's strong arm. I was relieved to finally get to bed at John's house at 11:30 p.m. It had been a long and very satisfying day. This was normal life again, and I may have still looked like a Cancer patient, but on the inside, I knew that I was not still a Cancer patient. My life had begun again.

Easter dawned cold and wet. The temperature was down into the high thirties. Everyone's new spring Easter outfits were inappropriate with this winter weather. Paul and I went to church with John in his new Catholic home church. After church, we went to a big family dinner with John's wife's family (the Daboub clan). The food was good, and the company was most enjoyable. It was a nice place to celebrate the end of my Cancer.

Sunday evening, the diarrhea hit. It continued throughout the week. My knee pain got better. I worked on the Grapevine house, visited with friends, went to the dentist, and generally took care of errands and jobs. We actually did a little entertaining in Grapevine this time. We hosted our neighbors, Bob and Marilyn Gunn, on Monday evening, after seeing *The Alamo* together. We hosted our good friends, Mary Lee and Frank Hamisch, on Wednesday evening. It was fun to get back into our normal routine of having folks over for dinner. We hadn't done much of that in the last year.

On Friday, April 16, we loaded up Mr. Pye and returned to Houston. We stopped in Conroe, had dinner with our old friends, Linda Lou and Miles McDonald, and then spent the night in Spring with Jeff and Liz so that we could stay with our granddaughter Erica while her parents went out together. We got back to our little apartment, our Houston home, on Monday, April 19.

Quitting Lexapro

I decided to stop taking my antidepressant pills cold turkey. I had taken 20 mg. of Lexapro throughout my year with Cancer. When I stopped taking the Lexapro, each evening, I had trouble getting my sleeping habits and patterns back. I hadn't realized that all of the wonderful sleep that I had gotten during my Cancer year was thanks to Lexapro. I began to think that Lexapro might even have been the cause for all of the happy, vivid dreams that I enjoyed. I found that now I struggled some to make my nights restful and good. But I was determined to wean myself from as many drugs as I could. My chemo was now over, and I should be strong enough emotionally to handle my problems.

Healing from Final Treatment

I was healing. I had been fighting diarrhea now for over a week. My nails had stopped dying. They stopped their oozing and seemed to be settling down. They actually seemed to be growing again. I was fighting mouth sores. I was also drinking cranberry juice a lot and was supplementing with cranberry pills. I wanted to try to avoid my usual bladder infection after each FAC treatment. A nurse in the Breast Center had finally told me that Cytoxan (the *C* drug in FAC) was especially harsh on a woman's bladder. The neuropathy in my feet remained a continual nagging problem, hindering my walking and certainly my stability. I was going through the side effects of the last chemo treatment, but this was the last time that I had to do it.

Slowly my hair started growing back all over my body. I had fuzz on my arms and legs now. The hair on my head grew in quickly, and soon I again had a good one-fourth inch of fuzz. It looked like it was coming in salt and pepper (gray, black, and white). My eyebrows grew in very quickly and were very black. My skin looked nearly normal all over my body, except on my arms. My arms still had the splotches and blots from the chemo sores. I was very hopeful that they would quickly lighten and eventually disappear. I looked better now. I did not look so much like a "Cancer" patient anymore. I was getting stronger each day. I knew now that I would recover from the treatments of Cancer. However, I knew that I would never be the same as I was at the beginning of 2003. *Cancer had definitely left its mark.*

I wanted to enjoy life. I wanted to pick and choose what I spent my time doing. I didn't want to do any more "hospital" things. I had realized the extreme value of having "friends." I could have never fought this battle without my "friends," family, and Paul. I knew that I would be all right. God had helped me through this, and I prayed that I would never have to experience Cancer again. In fact, I prayed that I would not have to die sick. I never wanted to be sick again.

Chapter 36

NORMAL LIFE IS GOOD

Normal Life Wasn't Easy

Because we wanted to stay in Houston through the "hangover" time of this last chemo treatment, we did not move back to Grapevine immediately. We wanted to stay close to MD Anderson until I had fully recovered from the effects of this last treatment. Hopefully, we had learned our lesson about *staying close to my doctors*. As badly as we wanted to pick up and to go home immediately, we stayed in our apartment in Houston.

Normal life was returning. It was grand, but there were days when I wondered if I was really ready for a full life again. I had been accustomed to the protected stay-in hibernation lifestyle that I had lived all through my Houston stay. This "normal" life nearly ran me ragged some days. We returned from our Easter trip to the DFW area and immediately started preparing for our move back home to Grapevine. I packed the "nonurgent" stuff, and we began living in an apartment with boxes stacked all around. It was like living in limbo or never-never land. Things seemed quite strange.

Good-bye to Houston

We finally set about to say good-bye to our Houston friends. I made my last trip to MD Anderson on April 22 for my last counseling session. I said good-bye to all of the people who worked in the Breast Center. The receptionists and the volunteers had become my friends over the last few months. I even hunted down and met the young man who acted as my phone interface to MD Anderson in the very beginning of my adventures there. I said good-bye to my nurse friends and my counselor. Everyone at MD Anderson knows that when you finally leave, it is a good thing. However, everyone has mixed emotions in that you are leaving "old" friends.

I got all of my medical reports and records, met with the financial people, and rode my bike home on the Braes Bayou trail one last time. The bright sunflowers had grown to be about eight feet tall now and bordered the trail with yellow and brown blossoms. The sun was shining brightly, and I was glad to know that my ordeal was finally over. I had taken the "unplanned journey" and would soon be going home to family and friends that I had known in happier times.

On Friday, April 23, we loaded up the back of the pickup with our table and four of our chairs, my comfy, soft lounge chair, the file cabinets that I had bought to give us drawer space in our closet, the three big end tables that had served us so well in our living room, and lots of little odds and ends. These were the things that I had bought from garage sales to furnish our apartment that I did not want to haul back to Grapevine. I planned to sit out in a vacant lot the next morning (Saturday) and sell these things garage-sale style. To my sorrow, we woke up early Saturday morning with the alarm to discover that it was pouring down rain outside. My garage sale plans were kaput. We lived in an apartment complex behind locked gates. I could never hold a garage sale in this place. Since I had taken a cold on Thursday and didn't feel really well anyway, we turned off the alarm, rolled over, and just slept in. I would never have been able to be that lazy before I had Cancer. I was an *A* personality and would push and push until I got things done. Cancer had made me more relaxed. I had learned to just *"let the chips fall where they will, and don't fight the small stuff."*

About 1:00 p.m., the sky started to clear, and it stopped raining. We got into our truck and immediately drove over to the Bluebonnet Shop. This was a charity resale shop that takes your merchandise, prices it, displays it for three months, and if it doesn't sell, starts reducing the price until it does sell. You will get 60 percent of the selling price if it is sold before the ninety days. If it doesn't sell in the ninety-day period, you just automatically donate it to the shop and only get a tax deduction. Since I couldn't sell our unwanted furniture in a garage sale, we figured that this was a good option. We did not want to try to move it back to Grapevine.

One should notice that I went all the way through this chemotherapy from October until April without ever taking a bad cold. Then as soon as I was nearly done, I took one. I had been very lucky through my treatments in not having to deal with another illness—the common cold. I felt bad for four days and did a lot of lying around and sleeping, but I got through the cold without any complications. I guess that colds are a part of a normal life, so in that way, I suppose that I should be thankful.

Final Activities

We said good-bye to all of our church friends at Salem Lutheran Church (our Houston church home) on Sunday, April 25. This group of people opened their arms and welcomed us into their fellowship, and it was sweet. We will forever hold a warm spot in our hearts for this little church, its pastor, and its people.

That evening we went to an Astro baseball game, where a guy in the stands ran out on the field and flashed his bare bottom. We went to my Aunt Eunice's memorial service in Bangs a small town near Colemant, TX., driving and returning in one day. Aunt Eunice was 99¾ years of age. She had been in a rest home in Albuquerque for several years, suffering with Alzheimer's. Her death was a blessing. It was really nice seeing a lot of my cousins, my mother, and my sister at this affair. Karen, my sister, hosted a sandwich luncheon in Coleman after the service, and we all got together and visited. This was the first time that I had seen this part of my family since I knew that I had Cancer. It was a nice reunion.

Houston in Our Rearview Mirror

Thursday morning, April 29, we had planned to get up and to finish the last-minute packing. However, we woke up to find that Paul had a very bad cold and an extremely sore throat, which might be a strep throat infection. Instead of packing, I ended up hunting a clinic that would see Paul that morning. We didn't have a general doctor in Houston so it was a bit of a job to get him in on such short notice. However, I got it done. We were able to see a nurse practitioner who looked at Paul and prescribed Allegra, a decongestant, and an antibiotic. I hoped that Paul could make a very speedy recovery because we were moving that afternoon. This unexpected illness really threatened our move plans. Paul was unable to work much and might even be contagious. What a mess! Neither of us wanted to postpone the move so I proceeded on assuring Paul that I would just do the move.

Our good friends, Marlene and Dick Van Horne, whom we had known for many years in Grapevine, arrived at our door at the precise preplanned time of 2:00 p.m. Peter and Jeff, our Houston sons, called and had moved their arrival times to 4:00 p.m. because of business appointments. We explained our problems to Marlene and Dick and gave them the option of escaping. They braved the storm, however, and opted to dig in and to help us pack and move. How badly we needed them that day!

Marlene started right in to finish the packing in the kitchen. Dick and I went out and hooked our pickup to our trailer and moved it around into the "moving spot" in our complex, which was approximately 130 to 160 yards from our apartment door. We began hauling out boxes and junk to the trailer. Paul could not help much; he was just too sick. When Peter and Jeff arrived, we moved the bed and the heavy things. About 6:00 p.m., much to my amazement, we had the trailer pretty well loaded. Everyone was exhausted and left with our great gratitude to return to their own homes. Peter stayed for a while and we took him to dinner. I got to eat the delicious raw Gulf Coast oysters that I had not been able to eat while I was fighting Cancer. My oncologist's orders had been to eat no raw fish or meat during chemo treatments. I loved these oysters and had not been able to enjoy them for the last six months. This was a real sign that chemo and Cancer were over.

We had planned to spend the night at Peter's house since we had no bed now, but since Paul was sick, we decided that we had better stay at our empty apartment and not expose Peter's children to Paul's bad cold. We slept that night on a single mattress on the floor and in our recliner chair. It wasn't a good night, but we got through it.

We only had last-minute little things to pack up on Friday morning, but it took us until 1:30 p.m. to get everything loaded, to clean the apartment, and to check out. We loaded Mr. Pye (our cat) into the car with me and pulled out. Paul drove the pickup truck, with the truck packed with our bikes, our clothes in wardrobe boxes, and other stuff. He pulled the trailer, and I followed in our loaded Camry. We were glad to say good-bye to Houston. All of the individual people that we met in Houston were *really* nice. I don't think we met anyone who wasn't friendly and kind. However, when you put the people together into the city, it just wasn't good. It was good to get Houston in our "rearview mirror" for the final time.

My Last Cancer Report

Life was returning to normal. Cancer was receding into the background. My fingernails were growing longer every day. Soon my thumbnails covered the end of my thumbs. The other fingernails already just about came to the end of my fingers. They were no longer oozing and dying. My two big toenails seemed to be growing a little. The hair that I started growing in March had all fallen out. It had gotten to be about three-eighths of an inch long and was very fine and thin (almost like baby's hair). In early May, my scalp started feeling "funny" again. The longer hair just disappeared after my last chemo treatment, and a thick short crop of new hair appeared. I hoped that this hair would be permanent. It seemed to be growing slower than the first hair did, but it was much thicker and sturdier. It appeared to be white or blond. I did have some eyebrows (not enough, but a few). I had some fuzz on my arms now.

The only bad thing that I had left from the Cancer was the neuropathy that I had in the front of my feet—my toes. My steps were not sure and firm like they used to be. I would not be sure-footed again until I got the feeling back into my toes.

Making the Wishes Come True

Cancer was gone, and life was back to "normal." It was a beautiful spring. I was in the process of decluttering and remodeling our Grapevine house. What a job! It took me fifteen years to get it this messed up, and it was going to take me several years to get it unmessed. I knew that I mustn't get impatient. Life was good, and Paul and I were very lucky.

Mr. Pyewacken (Mr. Pye) is a fabulous cat and a super companion. We are sorry that Mr. Boots left us soon after we arrived in Houston but are happily blessed in his absence with Mr. Pye. I will write Mr. Pye's story and describe the wonderful help and comfort that he gave me during my chemo in a later book or article. I call him my "God's Gift" kitty.

We returned to Colorado that summer. I grew lots of dark brown curly hair. The blotches on my skin went away, and I was beautiful (at least as beautiful as an old fat lady can be) again. My grandchildren grew, and we welcomed more into the family. I now have nineteen delightful, loving grandchildren who give me tons of pleasure, entertainment, and joy. My strength has returned, and I am healthy. I went this year, 2009, for my five-year checkup and got a good report from my oncologist, Dr. Brawn.

The physical facilities of MD Anderson have changed a lot since I was there fighting my Cancer, but the helpful, caring atmosphere hasn't changed at all. I still see lots of really sick people there who look like they have Cancer. With each one that I see, I say a silent prayer of thanks that I do not have that disease now. The Cancer monster (the fear that I will have Cancer again) always lurks in the dark just behind me, but so far, I have been able to stay ahead of it.

I am very busy and I often remember the promise that I made to God in the early spring and late winter of 2004, when I was so tired and so bored during my Chemo. *I promised that if I could just get through this horrible time, I would never again fuss about "being too busy."* I love my life.

My soapbox speech is to tell everyone that I can how important it is to do their monthly self-breast exams. I tell a much shortened version of my finding "the lump" experience when a doctor's exam and a mammogram did not find it. I want everyone to understand that a mammogram is a super diagnostic tool, and we all need regular mammograms, but all Cancers do not show up on a mammogram. One *must* do regular self-breast exams. It is super important to find Cancer early.

I am trying to make the things that I listed that I would have if I conquered my bad thing (my Cancer) come true on the back of the board that I broke on August 7, 2003, just before my boob burst. I didn't really take any time to think about these wishes when I wrote them down, but now that I have completed the unplanned journey, I think it is important to see whether these wishes are coming true in my life. I will always treasure this little piece of wood that I managed to break with my left hand. I display the board proudly in our home on a stand on our bookshelves in our living room. It is a constant reminder to me of what I accomplished. Those things (or wishes) that I felt like I could accomplish after I conquered Cancer were "love for all, health, strength, energy, new opportunities, a book, and possibilities." I think that I am fulfilling them in the following ways:

1. <u>Love for all</u>. I try to tell everyone that I love them. Before I say good-bye on the phone to any of my friends or family, I always say very quickly, "I love you. Good-bye." I try to find an excuse to tell people that I love them in my conversations. I think that I sometimes embarrass people with these words, but I think that this is an important phrase to say, "I love you." In doing this, I hope that I am making my wish that I made on the back of the board come true.

BREAST CANCER: THE UNPLANNED JOURNEY - LESSONS LEARNED

2. <u>Health</u>. I am finally healthy again, and I work to stay that way by exercising regularly, taking my prescribed medicines (Aromasin and Crestor) and my health pills (vitamin, fish oil, Glucosamine with Chondroitin, an aspirin, and calcium), seeing the doctor regularly, and trying to live happily.

3. <u>Strength</u>. I try to remain strong even though it gets harder as I get older (I am now sixty-seven). I walk and exercise regularly to keep my body strong. I attend church regularly in an effort to keep my spirit strong. I read and write to keep my mind strong.

4. <u>Energy</u>. Sometimes my energy levels are low, but I work hard to keep up. Most people are impressed with my energy levels. I try never to let a sore knee or other ache or pain keep me from getting up and working and going. I am not ready to be "handicapped."

5. <u>New opportunities</u>. I try to always be open to new opportunities, and I am not afraid to have new adventures. I went back to snow skiing, even though my toes were numb. I still enjoy a couple of months of downhill skiing in the winter. I love the freedom, the wind blowing in my face, and the sheer excitement of flying down a mountain of white. I began to play the keyboard in a jazz band. I also became the pianist for one of our church services. I climbed the bridge in the harbor at Sydney, Australia. I white-water rafted in New Zealand and even got out of the boat to go down one rapid just in my wet suit. I think that I am nearly always willing to try new things.

6. <u>A book</u>. The book that came out of my Cancer you are now reading, *Breast Cancer: The Unplanned Journey—Lessons Learned*. The writing of this book has been a journey in itself for me. I began the book in the fall of 2004, but I just couldn't write it at that time. When I would start to write, I couldn't see the computer screen because my vision would be clouded so by the tears that were streaming down my face. I just could not go through the experience again that quickly. However, in 2006, I was ready to write, and in December 2009, I finished the first manuscript. I have since edited my writings. In 2011, I got brave enough to take the next step to get it professionally edited and then to seek a publisher. Writing the book was a cleansing experience for me. I had to get my feelings and thoughts together to be able to write what I felt. I have been completely honest in my feelings in this book. I was not honest with my feelings when I was going through the unplanned journey.

7. <u>Possibilities</u>. This wish was probably an expression of the desire to know the future, and I don't have insights into that. However, my life continues to change all of the time. Hopefully, I will always be strong enough and open enough to change with life's demands. This year, it has been my job to take on new responsibilities in our married life as Paul's health deteriorates, and we are learning to live with his beginning dementia. Hopefully, I am living the possibilities that come into my life each day with grace.

This manuscript is the filling of "a book" wish. I now think that after I have completed this book, I have several other books to write. I hope to start my next book as soon as this one is finished. I need to work on getting a final manuscript out on my *Flat Stanley* children's books before I write the other book that now germinates in my brain. Thank you very much for following me through *Breast Cancer: The Unplanned Journey*. It was quite a trip. It was the most difficult thing that I have done in my life. I hope that it changed me for the better, and I hope that reading about my journey and the things that I learned from Cancer helps you get through your journeys.

Lessons Learned

1. Friends would turn out to be very valuable resources for encouragement and strength when I battled Cancer. (Chapter 1)
2. Facing the worst makes the problem seem smaller. (Chapter 1)
3. Everything moves so slowly. (Chapter 2)
4. Nothing moved as quickly as I would have liked. My life was filled all along the way with many hours of waiting. (Chapter 2)
5. Make the journey one step at a time. I had to do one simple thing at time. (Chapter 3)
6. Please be there in person for your friends who go through similar experiences, even if they tell you that they don't need you. (Chapter 3)
7. I had to accept the fact that I had Cancer, and I had to somehow go on. (Chapter 3)
8. Ask questions and find answers. Facts served to better arm me for the fears and trials ahead. (Chapter 4)
9. Use other's support, but watch out for the negative. (Chapter 5)
10. I decided that it was best if I didn't truthfully answer all questions. Casual friends don't really want to know how you are when you are dealing with a devastating diagnosis of Cancer. (Chapter 5)
11. Life and plans go on. Go with the flow. (Chapter 6)
12. One should not get behind the pain curve. (Chapter 6)
13. Follow the doctor's directions, especially with pain management. (Chapter 7)
14. Being honest about my pain was not always good, but I needed to learn to be more open with my partner. (Chapter 7)
15. You can't "tough it out" with Cancer. (Chapter 7)
16. Carefully keep your records—medical and personal. (Chapter 8)
17. Find good models—Cancer survivors. (Chapter 9)
18. Store memories of strength and happiness. (Chapter 10)
19. Listen to your body. (Chapter 11)

BREAST CANCER: THE UNPLANNED JOURNEY - LESSONS LEARNED

20. Cancer is not a disease for sissies! (Chapter 11) Only the tough, positive people survive Cancer. (Chapter 13)
21. I shouldn't ever really leave the area where my doctor was located. (Chapter 11)
22. Patience—fighting cancer is not a race. (Chapter 12)
23. The journey can be full of unexpected turns—just go on. (Chapter 13)
24. Be prepared to submit to and perform all kinds of medical procedures. (Chapter 13)
25. A decision-making committee is a necessity. (Chapter 14)
26. Keep reminders of love and support with you. (Chapter 15)
27. It gets darkest just before the dawn. (Chapter 17)
28. Cancer is a disease that I could not beat by myself. I needed lots of support. (Chapter 17)
29. Study how other people have successfully beaten Cancer. (Chapter 18)
30. Inner-mind symbols reflect your life. (Chapter 18)
31. Communicate your inner fears and feelings. (Chapter 18)
32. You are never completely done with Cancer. (Chapter 18)
33. Use successful Cancer survivors to model your own life from. (Chapter 18)
34. Life goes on, and I would go on with it (even if I had to fight Cancer on the journey). (Chapters 18 and 19)
35. Knowledge helped to dispel those monsters that crept up in hard times. (Chapter 18)
36. In the general population, one out of every three people will have Cancer today. One of every eight women will have breast Cancer. Cancer is a fact of life today. (Chapter 18)
37. Cancer is a chronic disease rather than a terminal disease. It is often curable. (Chapter 18)
38. Cancer seems to break down the walls between strangers so that immediately you are friends. (Chapter 19)
39. Take advantage of any sabbatical time that you have. See your friends and family. Rest your mind and body so that your spirit can be strengthened. Use every moment, and don't waste any of the "good" time. The battle lies ahead and may be difficult. (Chapter 19)
40. Gather your support team and use them often. (Chapter 20)
41. Talk about your innermost thoughts and fears. (Chapter 22)
42. Remember the important things. (Chapter 23)
43. When you reach the bottom of the hole, there is no way to go but up. (Chapter 24)
44. Get your prayer support team and all your friends engaged anytime that you need them. (Chapter 25)
45. Looking back on the earlier "hard times" in my life, I could see that they weren't really as bad as I had earlier thought they were. (Chapter 26)

46. Anyone facing Cancer should seek out counseling help so that you can discuss your private and inner fears and thoughts. (Chapter 27)
47. Quantifying the time involved in finishing a difficult task seems to make it easier to accomplish. (Chapter 28)
48. Be with your family for pleasant times as much as you can. (Chapter 29)
49. I have never heard of anyone not growing their hair back after chemo. It will be okay again sometime. (Chapter 29)
50. Don't ever be too proud to accept caring people's support. (Chapter 29)
51. Let your smile be your shield against Cancer. (Chapter 29)
52. People with Cancer enjoy the simple things—a short, sweet conversation, a child's smile, a lovely flower, and a hug. (Chapter 29)
53. Work to be "bald and beautiful." (Chapter 29)
54. Thank God for all of your wonderful family and friends who help you through hard times. (Chapter 30)
55. Use the good days to keep you going through the bad days. (Chapter 30)
56. Breast Cancer is the scourge of the devil, if ever there is one. (Chapter 30)
57. Thank God for the ability to sleep. (Chapter 30)
58. Your Cancer battle takes time and must be fought one day at a time. (Chapter 30)
59. Please remember that a bad hair day is better anytime than a no-hair day. (Chapter 31)
60. I could be sad and cry this year because of the many things that I cannot do or have, but I choose to be as happy as I can and to enjoy the blessings that come my way instead. (Chapter 31)
61. Learn to be patient and quiet. (Chapter 31)
62. Cancer is a powerful and dreadful disease that affects everyone around in an unforgettable way. (Chapter 33)
63. Don't forget to always count your blessings. (Chapter 33)
64. Don't criticize anyone else for doing something that seems to be stupid. You don't know how they feel unless you have walked in their shoes. Be understanding of others now even when what they do seem crazy. (Chapter 34)
65. This (time of chemo) too shall pass. (Chapter 34)
66. Chemo does strange things to your sense of smell and taste. (Chapter 34)
67. Cancer is curable if found early. (Chapter 34)
68. Chemo has to be the worst "good" thing that you can do to your body. (Chapter 34)
69. I held fast to the fact that each day near my apartment, the bayou kept running to the sea and the sun kept rising and setting, and I knew that I too would continue on this road that I had started (chemo), although it certainly was something that I really did not want to do.
70. Love is the grease that keeps the life machine going. (Chapter 34).

BREAST CANCER: THE UNPLANNED JOURNEY - LESSONS LEARNED

71. Friends are one of the sweetest things in life. (Chapter 35)
72. And oh, how *sweet* life is (after Cancer)! I am very happy to be alive and to *not* have Cancer in my body. (Chapter 35)
73. Cancer had definitely changed me. (Chapter 35)
74. Let the chips fall where they will, and don't fight the small stuff. (Chapter 36)
75. I promised God that if I could just get through this horrible time, I would never again fuss about "being too busy." (Chapter 36)

Edwards Brothers, Inc.
Thorofare, NJ USA
February 28, 2012